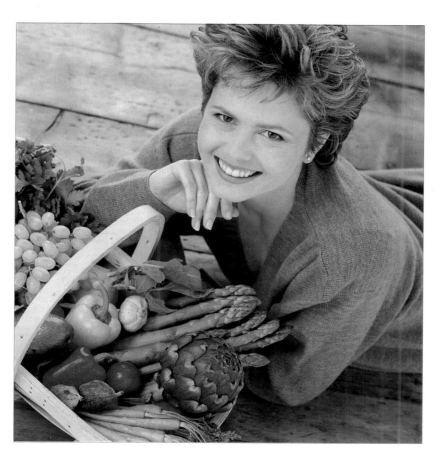

Liz Earle's
LIFESTYLE GUIDE

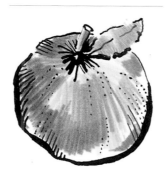

Liz Earle's
LIFESTYLE GUIDE

The complete system of nutrients, activities and beauty
techniques for a healthier lifestyle

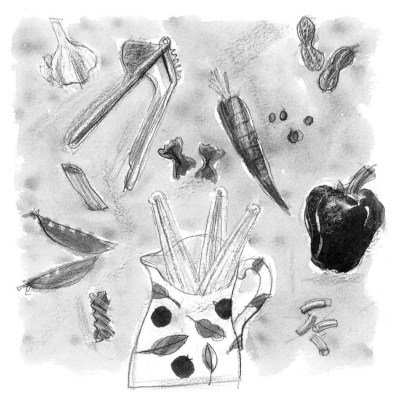

B⬥XTREE

ADVICE TO THE READER

Before following any medical or dietary advice contained in this book, it is recommended that you consult your doctor if you suffer from any health problems or special conditions or are in any doubt as to its suitability.

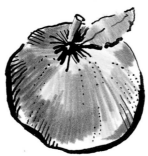

Published in Great Britain in 1995 for The Boots Company PLC by Boxtree Limited, Broadwall House, 21 Broadwall, London SE1 9PL

Copyright (c) Liz Earle 1995

The right of Liz Earle to be identified as Author of this work has been asserted by her in accordance with the Copyright, Designs and Patents Act 1988

1 3 5 7 9 10 8 6 4 2

ISBN 0 7522 0501 3

Designed by Hammond Hammond
Cover design by Newell and Sorrell Limited and Major, Taylor, Nicholson
Illustrations by Angelika Elsebach
Typesetting by Michael Weintroub

Printed and bound in Italy by New Interlitho Spa.

A CIP catalogue entry for this book is available from the British Library

CONTENTS

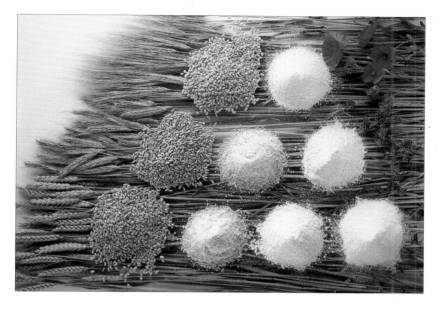

ACKNOWLEDGEMENTS

I am grateful to many who have helped with the research and preparation of this book, especially my editorial assistant Sarah Hamilton-Fleming. I would also like to express my sincere thanks to several healthcare professionals for their invaluable expertise, notably Dr Ann Walker, Lecturer in Human Nutrition at the University of Reading, and Rhonda Smith at the charity Research Into Ageing. I am also grateful for the support and practical help given by Jan Petherick and her team at Cameron Choat & Partners. Thanks also to the talented Terence Renati, hairdresser and photographer, for the back jacket photograph. Last, but by no means least, my thanks to the capable and talented team at Boxtree for making this project possible.

INTRODUCTION

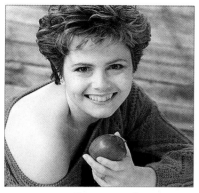

We must all now be aware of the need for a much greater understanding about our general lifestyles. Our changing environment has placed us all under an increasing amount of tension and strain. Our diet is also rapidly changing and we are eating foods that are drastically different to those of our parents' and grandparents' generations. The rise in processed and 'junk' foods has led to a poorly nourished nation in need of nutritional nurturing. Fortunately, new research has shown that there are many beneficial nutrients in the form of vitamins and minerals. The key is to understand which nutrients can help us at the various stages of our lives. Whether we are nine, nineteen or ninety there are many simple lifestyle changes that can help us all strengthen our health and enable us to cope more easily with modern living. This book sets out many of the stages of your life and describes how to take positive action to enhance your physical well-being – no matter what your age. I sincerely hope that it will help you in the same way that the information it contains has dramatically improved my own life, and that of my family.

I wish you the very best of health.

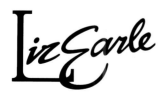

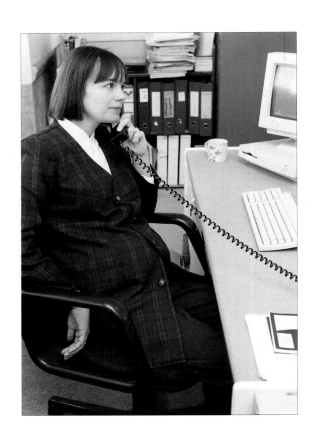

1

Busy

M odern life means that we have never been busier or had so many demands placed on our time. Many of us have to juggle the needs of our family, career and personal relationships while trying to beat stress and stay fit, attractive and healthy. This takes a great deal of effort and hard work which consume our energy stores, often leaving us feeling tired, devitalised and prone to developing colds and other minor ailments. However, the good news is that we do not have to feel this way, no matter how many demands are made on us. It is possible for everyone, young or old, to boost their energy levels, support the immune system and promote all-round health by adopting a varied diet supplying the nutrients we need to function successfully under pressure. In this introductory chapter, we look at the principles of healthy eating and find out how diet and supplements can help nervous tension and stress. There is also advice on how to incorporate relaxation techniques and exercise into a busy schedule, as well as a selection of my favourite quick and easy beauty treats to boost the body beautiful.

EATING FOR HEALTH
In any guide to healthy living, one of the first considerations must be what we put into our bodies. Food is our life source – without it we will die. But it is important to eat the right foods if we wish to live long and active lives. To maintain energy levels and optimum health, our diet should be a well-balanced mixture of natural foods, including fish, wholegrains, fruits, vegetables, oils and herbs. These are high energy foods, rich in the

nutrients our bodies need. At the other end of the scale are the low-energy foods, such as 'junk foods', which tend to be high in saturated fat and sugar, and processed foods, which almost always contain additives and preservatives. These products often have very little nutritional value, so although the occasional take-away pizza or ready-made lasagne won't do any damage, they should not be a daily part of our diet.

The healthy eating guidelines outlined in this chapter tally with the Government's *Health of the Nation* report. There is a clear link between a high intake of saturated fat and the increased risk of cancer, heart disease and other degenerative diseases, and this report calls for a reduction in the percentage of daily calories we get from total fat (down from about 40 percent in 1990 to no more than 35 percent by the year 2005). It also advises a reduction in the percentage of calories derived from saturated fat (from 17 percent in 1990 to no more than 11 percent by 2005).

To improve our all-round health and help protect our body, we should follow these healthy eating guidelines, which also form the basis for maintaining a slim, fit figure. (News for dieters will be covered in Chapter 3).

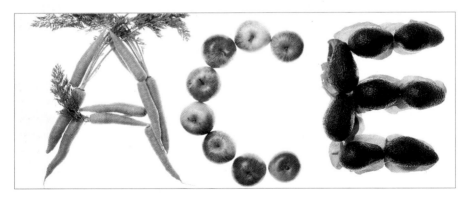

HEALTHY EATING GUIDELINES

In addition to a little protein such as meat, fish and eggs, and dairy products (in moderation), try to eat the following foods every day:

Wholegrains	2 or more types
Fresh fruit	2 or more varieties
Vegetables	3 or more varieties
Vegetable oils	1 dessertspoonful
Herbs and spices	2 or more types

WHOLEGRAINS Wholegrains are amazingly concentrated sources of protein, carbohydrate, fibre, vitamins and minerals – in fact, everything the body needs for creating vigour and energy. In their natural state, i.e. brown rice, wholewheat, millet, pot barley, buckwheat, maize, oats and rye, they are highly nutritious. Unfortunately, the modern diet consists mainly of refined grains in the form of white bread, pasta and polished rice. This means we may be missing out on many of the minerals and trace elements, such as calcium, potassium, magnesium, zinc and iron, that wholegrains contain.

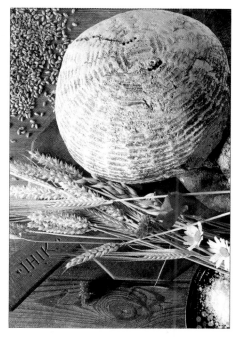

Calcium is needed to form healthy teeth and bones and it is found in dairy products and leafy vegetables. **Potassium** is involved in energy production. It also ensures the removal of excess sodium and therefore may have a role in helping to prevent high blood pressure. It also helps prevent water retention. The best sources of potassium are wheat bran, bananas, fresh orange juice and dried fruits. **Magnesium** is needed to enable the vitamins B1 (thiamine), which is involved in energy production, and B6 to function properly. Low levels of B6 can result in depression. Magnesium is also needed for protein metabolism and energy production, and those on high protein diets should ensure that they are getting enough of this mineral. It helps to maintain healthy body cells and is expelled from the body through sweat, so those who enjoy plenty of sport need to get a regular supply. Nuts, legumes (such as peanuts and pulses) and wholegrains are the richest sources of magnesium.

Zinc is essential for normal growth and it promotes rapid healing of wounds. It also aids the development of the reproductive organs. The best sources of zinc are seafood, beef, cheese and wholemeal bread. **Iron** is an important oxygen carrier in the blood and forms an essential part of the enzymes and the immune substances necessary to destroy invading organisms. Iron deficiency is especially common in women who do not eat much meat. If this applies to you, it may be worth taking an iron supplement. The best sources of iron are liver, kidney, all types of meat, spinach, wholemeal bread and fortified breakfast cereals.

Wholegrains are rich sources of all these minerals and trace elements, much more so than their refined counterparts, such as white bread, white pasta and white rice. Refined white flour contains about a fifth of the magnesium and zinc content of wholemeal flour and has less than a quarter of the vitamin E content (an important antioxidant – more about this later). Refined flour is also remarkably low in fibre. Wholegrains, on the other hand are good fibre providers and so help our bodies to eliminate waste more effectively. Wholegrain breakfast cereals supply about ten times as much fibre as ordinary cornflakes, so a simple switch in cereal can significantly boost our fibre intake.

FRESH FRUIT Fruits are an important source of vitamins, minerals and enzymes and their high fibre and water content make them a wonderful internal cleanser. The fibre in fruit helps to bind with toxins and impurities in the body and assists their removal, while the water gently flushes these impurities out of the system. Fruit fibre is also easier to digest than wheat bran and is low in calories too.

Fruit is one of the best sources of the antioxidants vitamin C and beta-carotene. Antioxidants help prevent damage to our cells by free radicals. An excess of free radicals is now widely thought to be linked to cancer, heart disease and many other degenerative diseases. The World Health Organisation recommend we eat five servings of fruit and/or vegetables (excluding potatoes) every single day.

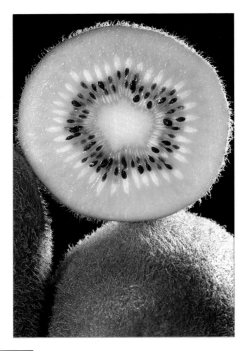

Fruits are most beneficial when they are eaten raw as they contain valuable enzymes that trigger a huge range of chemical reactions within the body. Enzymes perish when exposed to air and so fruit is best eaten as soon as it is cut. Nutrient values also begin to diminish as soon as the fruit has been picked and some fruits, such as oranges, may be stored for many months before reaching the supermarket shelves. One way to ensure that the fruits you are buying are freshly harvested is to choose organically grown produce. Organic fruits and vegetables are not sprayed with preservatives, toxic insecticides or fungicides. They do not keep as well as those sprayed with preservatives, but this means that they are not stored for long before sale.

VEGETABLES Vegetables, like fruit, are rich in the fibre that cleanses our system and are the mainstay of any healthy eating regime. They are also rich in vitamins and minerals and contain the two main antioxidants vitamin C and beta-carotene. Try to have some kind of vegetable with each meal, even if it is only some dark lettuce leaves and a few slices of tomato in a sandwich. Nowadays there are a great many vegetables available throughout the year.

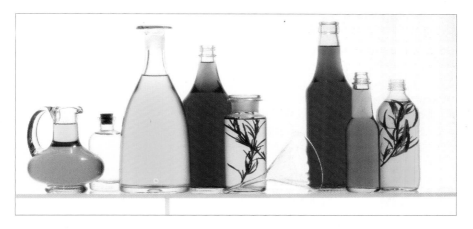

VEGETABLE OILS Oils are generally extracted from nuts, seeds and wholegrains. Plant oils, such as olive oil, are a rich source of vitamin E. Many large-scale clinical trials have indicated that vitamin E helps to protect us against heart disease. Vegetable and fish oils also contain nutrients known as essential fatty acids (EFAs), which are required by every living cell in the body in order to function properly. To emphasise the importance of EFAs the World Health Organisation advises that essential fatty acids should make up at least 3 percent of our total calorific intake; this should be increased to 5–6 percent for children and breast-feeding women.

Not all fat is so good for us – the saturated fat in meat and dairy products is actually bad for us if we eat too much of it. A diet that is high in saturates increases the 'bad' form of cholesterol that encourages deposits in the arteries and raises the risk of heart attacks and thrombosis. So, instead of cooking your food in butter, use olive oil and, instead of dolloping mayonnaise onto your salad, make a delicious dressing from olive oil and fresh lemon juice.

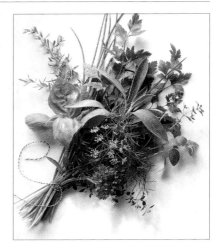

HERBS AND SPICES Herbs not only transform our food, they also have numerous health-giving properties. Modern medicine has yet to better many of Mother Nature's original healers, and the basis of most modern medicines lies in herbal remedies. By far the easiest way to reap the many benefits of herbs and spices is to make them part of your everyday meals. Many herbs have distinctive flavours which go particularly well with certain foods. Even some of the most common herbs used in cooking have powerful health-giving properties. Garlic, for example, helps to boost the immune system as well as helping to reduce blood cholesterol levels. Garlic capsules are sometimes taken to ward off cold and 'flu bugs.

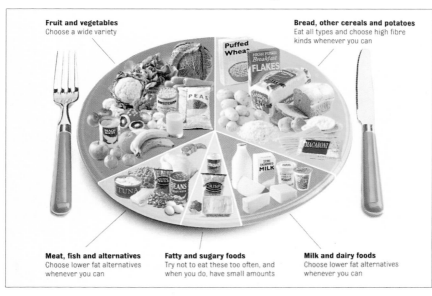

Fruit and vegetables
Choose a wide variety

Bread, other cereals and potatoes
Eat all types and choose high fibre kinds whenever you can

Meat, fish and alternatives
Choose lower fat alternatives whenever you can

Fatty and sugary foods
Try not to eat these too often, and when you do, have small amounts

Milk and dairy foods
Choose lower fat alternatives whenever you can

This guide to healthy eating can be easily represented in the form of a plate of food. As you can see, a third of the food plate is made up of complex carbohydrates (such as wholemeal bread and brown rice), which are our basic source of slow-release energy to keep us going throughout the day. Fresh fruit and vegetables should also feature highly in our diet and can be eaten as often as you like – aim to have at least five portions daily. Taking up less room on the food plate and therefore a smaller part of our diet, are protein foods such as meat, fish and their alternatives. The majority of us eat more protein than we need and we can obtain all the essential amino acids – the building blocks of protein – from a combination of vegetables, nuts, seeds, pulses or sprouts (we will come back to this in the following chapter on vegetarian food). It is also wise to keep a check on the amount of milk and dairy foods we eat as they can be high in saturated fat. Look for low-fat alternatives such as semi-skimmed milk and low-fat cheese and yoghurts. Finally, fatty and sugary foods should be eaten less often and in small quantities as they are high in calories and low in nutritional value.

FREE RADICALS AND ANTIOXIDANTS

Unfortunately, even if we have a perfectly healthy diet, we will be exposed to pollutants in the atmosphere, such as car exhaust fumes and cigarette smoke, which can adversely affect our health. In addition to car fumes, we are surrounded by many other invisible poisons including industrial pollutants such as cadmium, mercury and lead. These pollutants create an excess of free radicals, potentially destructive particles which attack our cells and may eventually lead to some kinds of cancer and heart disease. Unless you live in a bubble, it is impossible to avoid these pollutants, especially if you live in or near a town. Fortunately, the antioxidant nutrients can come to our rescue by neutralising many of the damaging free radicals.

The main antioxidants are vitamins A (in the form of beta-carotene), C and E and the mineral selenium. These are sometimes called the ACE vitamins. **Beta-carotene** is found in brightly coloured fruit and vegetables and is one important reason why we need to eat plenty of these. Apart from its antioxidant properties, **vitamin C** promotes iron absorption from food, helps to protect us against infection and may improve our resistance to bacteria and viral disease. **Vitamin E** is best known as an antioxidant that protects fatty tissues and cells in the body. The mineral **selenium** works with vitamin E as an antioxidant and also promotes normal growth and development.

Top-level research around the world shows that, in combination, these nutrients can provide us with the potential to boost our immunity to life-threatening illnesses, help prevent serious disorders, such as cataracts, and may even reduce signs of premature ageing, such as facial lines and wrinkles. Increased exposure to the UV rays of the sun also produces many more free radicals within the body, so we need to ensure we are getting ample supplies of antioxidants during the summer months or when on holiday abroad.

Copper and manganese are lesser known antioxidants. **Copper** is an essential component of many of the body's enzymes, including an enzyme that combats free radicals. It also forms part of the skin's proteins, collagen and elastin, and is important for maintaining a clear, smooth complexion. Liver, crab and hazelnuts are the best sources of copper. **Manganese** is part of the same antioxidant enzyme as copper and is also involved with the creation of interferon, an anti-viral and perhaps even anti-cancer compound agent, produced by the body in response to disease-producing viruses. Our best sources of manganese are wholegrain cereals and nuts and it is important to obtain a regular amount as we lose some of our manganese supply daily via excretion.

Experts suggest that we only need very small amounts of both copper and manganese, but we should be aiming for at least 12mg of beta-carotene, 100mg of vitamin C, 100mg of vitamin E and 150mcg of selenium. We can reach the desired levels of beta-carotene and vitamin C by eating at least five portions of fruit and vegetables each day (although, bear in mind that smoking, alcohol and caffeine all deplete our levels of vitamin C). We can also obtain the required amount of beta-carotene through eating five pieces of fruit or vegetables (excluding potatoes). If you do not eat this many fruit and vegetables every day, consider taking an antioxidant supplement.

Vitamin E is another case altogether, as it is not so widely available in foods. It can be found in wholemeal bread, wheatgerm and unrefined cooking oils, nuts and seeds, but you would need to eat 450g (1lb) of sunflower seeds, more than 2.5kg (5lb) of wheatgerm or drink over 2 litres (4 pints) of corn oil every day to achieve the same intake of vitamin E found in a common 268mg supplement. Selenium is even harder to obtain from the food we eat, but we must not underestimate its importance. Selenium can help protect us against cancer and heart disease and has the ability to boost the powers of other vitamins within the body. Selenium and vitamin E work synergistically and have a greater effect when taken together than on their own. Selenium is found in trace amounts in wholemeal flour, shrimps, strong white flour, crab, liver and kidney, but the levels of this important nutrient vary considerably depending upon selenium levels in the soil. Unfortunately, much of the grain we eat in this country comes from Europe and doesn't contain as much selenium as the hard wheat we used to import from Canada. The levels of selenium in British soil have also been dramatically reduced by intensive farming methods. It is therefore easier to get the selenium we need from a tablet or capsule.

It is particularly important for those who smoke to take an antioxidant supplement, (as smoking produces enormous amounts of free radicals) or better still, stop smoking altogether. It is estimated that in industrialised countries tobacco is now causing about 2 million deaths a year, killing at least a third of those who regularly smoke cigarettes. Smoking a cigarette is equivalent to force-feeding the body with free radicals, and cigarettes contain over forty known cancer-causing compounds. Smokers have lower levels of vitamin C in their bloodstream than non-smokers and studies show that smokers need to consume at least 150mg of vitamin C a day in order to achieve blood-levels of the vitamin comparable to those found in non-smokers.If you are a non-smoker but are exposed to cigarette smoke at home or work, it may be worth considering additional antioxidant supplies.

All four of these antioxidants (beta-carotene, vitamin C, vitamin E and selenium) are available together in supplement form and it may be more convenient to take a version that contains all four nutrients in one.

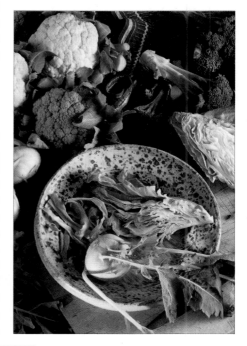

STRESS-BUSTING NUTRITION

The stresses of modern life can take their toll on the system, causing anything from general tiredness to digestive problems and frequent bouts of flu. An improved diet combined with relaxation and gentle exercise can help to combat these symptoms. The healthy eating guidelines previously outlined should boost your energy supplies and enable your body to cope better with stressful situations, such as exams, relationship difficulties or pressures at work. An antioxidant supplement will also help maintain your immune system, so that you are less likely to suffer from colds and flu.

Another supplement worth considering for stress is one containing the **B complex vitamins**. The B vitamins are B1 or thiamine (found in yeast extract, brown rice, nuts, pork and fortified breakfast cereals), B2 or riboflavin (found in milk, eggs, green leafy vegetables and lean meat), niacin (found in yeast extract, meat, oily fish, wholegrain cereals, dried fruit and dairy produce), B5 or pantothenic acid (found in yeast, nuts, offal, eggs and wholegrains), B6 or pyridoxine (found in wholemeal bread, wholewheat cereals, fortified breakfast cereals, liver, bananas, nuts and oily fish), folic acid (found in offal, green leafy vegetables, nuts, eggs, bananas, oranges and pulses) and B12 or cobalamin (found in offal, eggs, cheese, milk, meat and fish). They work synergistically – so are best taken together. As they are water soluble and are not stored by the body, we need a regular supply of them each day. Together, the B complex vitamins are essential for turning the food we eat into energy and low levels in our diet can lead to fatigue and even depression.

STRESS-BUSTING RELAXATION

To combat stress it is also important to take time out from our busy lives to concentrate on our own needs. Try to set some time aside each week, or perhaps for half an hour every day, which is devoted to yourself and nobody else. This might be on the train returning from work where you could read an interesting book; when the kids are sleeping or at school you can put your feet up and listen to some music (even if only for ten minutes), watch a programme on television that you particularly like, or you might prefer to paint or sing. Whatever it is you like to do, it should be relaxing and, while you do it, try to block from your mind all other considerations so that your mind and body are focused purely on the pleasurable activity.

BREATHING

The way in which we breathe can determine how effectively we eliminate toxins. In fact, more toxins are exhaled via the lungs than are passed through urine. For optimum health, we need to remove as many toxins as possible from our system. Instead of making use of our vast respiratory capacity, many of us walk or sit in a slumped position and are only using our upper chest when we breathe. If you adopt a healthier position, with head held high, back upright and shoulders back, good breathing should come naturally.

Here is a simple breathing exercise which will boost your energy levels and leave you feeling both relaxed and revived. Lie on the floor on your back somewhere away from distractions, preferably in the fresh air. Place a pillow under your knees and rest your hands on your abdomen above your navel. Take a long breath through your nose for three or four counts, and exhale slowly through your mouth for a count of four or five. Continue to breathe like this for at least five minutes and concentrate your mind solely on your breathing. You can do this exercise in the bath, while listening to music, in bed at night or in some other relaxed situation and it is a great way of relieving stress.

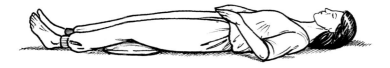

YOGA

Meditation, correct breathing and stretching are all involved in yoga which is a great way to tone and relax the body and calm the mind. Yoga helps us to release physical and mental tension, and our vast resources of energy. It is a complete science that encompasses body, mind and spirit. To achieve the renewed energy levels, fully toned body and peace of mind that yoga can induce, it is best to devote time to it each week. Below are some simple exercises that anyone can do to get themselves started (those who have back problems or other muscular problems should consult their GP beforehand).

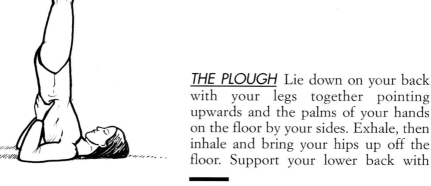

THE PLOUGH Lie down on your back with your legs together pointing upwards and the palms of your hands on the floor by your sides. Exhale, then inhale and bring your hips up off the floor. Support your lower back with your hands, keeping your elbows as close together as possible. Then, without bending your knees, exhale and bring your legs down behind your head. If your feet can't touch the floor, then remain in this position and breathe deeply. If they do comfortably reach the floor, then walk them up as close to your head as you can, with your toes touching the floor and your heels stretched back. Now clasp your hands together and stretch your arms out behind your back. Hold this position and breathe slowly and deeply.

THE BRIDGE Lie down on your back with your knees bent and feet together. Place your hands on your lower back and then lift your hips as high as you can. Then walk your legs out until your knees are straight and your feet flat on the floor. Hold the pose for at least three deep breaths, then walk your feet back in towards your body. Inhale, come into a shoulder stand and roll out.

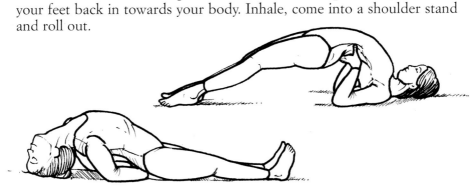

THE FISH Lie down on your back with your legs straight and your feet together. Lay your hands, palms down, underneath your thighs. Inhale as you press down on your elbows and arch your back, resting the very top of your head on the floor. Exhale. Breathe deeply while in this position and keep your legs and lower torso relaxed. To come out of the pose, raise your head and place it down, and then release your arms.

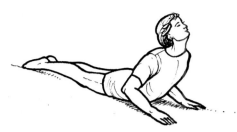
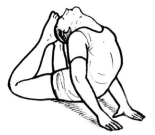

THE COBRA Lie down on your front with your legs together and the palms of your hands on the floor by your shoulders. Rest your forehead on the floor and inhale as you raise your head, brushing first your nose then your chin against the floor. Now lift up your hands and use your back muscles to raise your chest as far as possible from the ground. Hold for a few deep breaths and then return to the starting position. Repeat the stretch, but this time using your hands to push your chest up. Return to the initial position and repeat, this time again using your back muscles to lift your chest. To complete the position, walk your hands in towards your body, straighten your arms and lift your pelvis slightly. Then push out your chest, separate your legs, bend your knees, drop your head back and touch your head with your feet. Breathe normally and slowly return to the starting position.

MEDITATION We all seek the peace of mind that meditation brings and we all have our own methods of meditation, be it having a bath, knitting by the fire, or sitting in the sun. If while doing these activities, your thoughts concentrate on one object and your mind is fully absorbed in these relaxed thoughts, then you are meditating. It is possible to develop your ability to meditate, although at first your thoughts will insist on wandering. It is best to establish meditation as a regular habit of your life; something that you do at a particular time each day, as much a part of your routine as brushing your teeth.

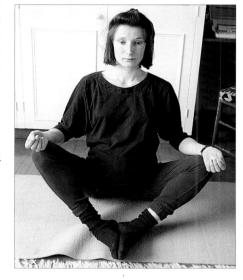

Choose a time of day when your mind is free from everyday concerns – dawn or dusk are usually best. Adopt a comfortable position from which to meditate, such as cross-legged or in the lotus position (see below). You may wish to wrap a blanket around you to keep warm. Then instruct your mind to be silent and to forget all thoughts, past, present or future. Regulate your breathing, close your eyes and concentrate your mind on one thought or image. This will relieve your mind of all the thousands of different thoughts, worries and anxieties that occupy it throughout the day, and help to induce a feeling of inner peace.

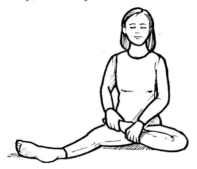 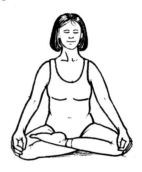

THE LOTUS Sit upright with your legs out in a 'V' shape in front of you. Bend one knee and bring the foot in, placing it high on the other thigh. Now bring the second foot in and place it under the opposite thigh to form the half lotus. For the full lotus, which is harder, you lift the second leg in over the first, placing the foot high on the opposite thigh.

THE BODY BEAUTIFUL

Having looked at the various ways we can relax our mind and body, restore energy levels and boost our health from the inside, it is now time to pay some attention to our protective outer shell: our skin. Taking time to bathe, massage and moisturise our skin is therapeutic for the mind as well as the body and leaves it glowing and healthy. I like to make my own beauty treatments from natural ingredients beneficial to the skin. Natural beauty care has played an important part in history. Recorded formulae for skin-softening lotions date back to Egyptian times, when women made lotions from the fragrant plant extracts to keep their skin smooth and supple.

SKIN BRUSHING

Before trying one of my favourite natural beauty recipes, it is worth removing all the grime and dead skin which lies on the very surface of the body. To do this, use either a coarse bristled body brush with a long handle, or a loofah. Start to brush from the tips of your fingers in long, firm strokes up your arms towards your shoulders. Then brush from your toes over and under your feet and up your shins and calves. Continue to brush from your knees up over your thighs. Home in on the tops of your thighs, brushing over your buttocks in towards your inner thighs in a circular motion. This is the main place where cellulite tends to develop and regular skin brushing can help to dislodge these ugly fat deposits by stimulating circulation and improving lymphatic drainage. Then brush up your lower back and sides and use a gentle circular movement over your tummy. Now you should start to brush down your neck, shoulders and upper back. Make sure you are always brushing towards your heart to stimulate blood circulation. Do not brush over areas of broken or inflamed skin or varicose veins. The whole process should only take a couple of minutes and you will feel a pleasant tingling sensation as the blood rushes to all your cells.

Skin brushing stimulates our circulation, bringing the blood to every part of the body to feed the cells with the nutrients it contains. Brushing also dislodges all the dead skin cells and grime that washing alone will not remove, leaving your skin clean and glowing with health. Now you can either have a bath or shower or try one of my beauty boosting recipes.

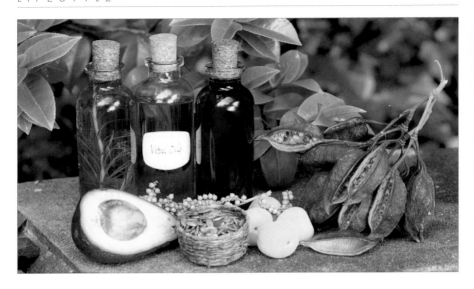

BODY TREATS

Extra-rich body lotion: This richly emollient skin lotion is excellent for the legs which have few sebaceous glands to keep them naturally moisturised. It is also good as an intensive hand cream or for smoothing skin on the elbows and knees.

50g (2oz) cocoa butter
30ml (2tbsp) calendula oil
15ml (1tbsp) avocado oil

5ml (1tsp) wheatgerm oil
10 drops chamomile, neroli or
* sandalwood essential oil*

Place the cocoa butter in a small saucepan and melt gently over a low heat. Remove from the stove and stir in the calendula, avocado and wheatgerm oils. Allow the mixture to cool before adding the chamomile essential oil. Pour into a large screw-top jar and apply liberally after bathing to dehydrated or chapped skin.

Anti-cellulite oil: This is no miracle cure for dimpled, 'orange-peel' thighs, but a blend used by aromatherapists to help the condition.

100ml (4fl oz) grapeseed oil
5ml (1tsp) wheatgerm oil
10 drops juniper essential oil

5 drops lemon essential oil
5 drops fennel essential oil

Mix all the oils together in a screw-top bottle or jar and shake well before use. Use daily on the hips and buttocks after bathing, massaging into the skin using firm, circular movements.

Remoisturising mask: Last, but not least, the face is exposed to the harsh elements of nature all year round and could do with some extra care and attention. This recipe is definitely not for eating as it is high in saturated fat and calories, but it does make a great moisturising mask! It contains lecithin, from the egg yolk, which helps to lock moisture into the skin. In addition, the buttermilk or yoghurt contains lactic acid, which is also an excellent moisturiser and with regular use can help to fade brown 'age' spots.

15ml (1tbsp) buttermilk
 or plain, live yoghurt
1 egg yolk

2.5ml ($^{1}\!/\!_{2}$tsp) honey
5ml (1tsp) mayonnaise

Mix all the ingredients together in a bowl until they form a smooth paste. Apply to clean, dry skin on the face and neck and leave for 15–20 minutes. Rinse thoroughly with plenty of warm water and pat dry.

A simpler version of this emollient mask may be made by mixing 2.5ml ($^{1}\!/\!_{2}$tsp) honey with one egg yolk. The honey forms a moisturising film on the face while the lecithin in the egg yolk is also deeply moisturising and helps bind moisture onto the skin's surface.

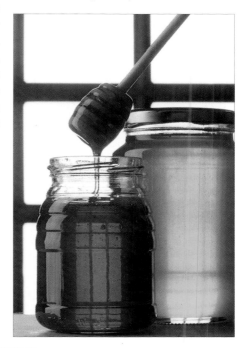

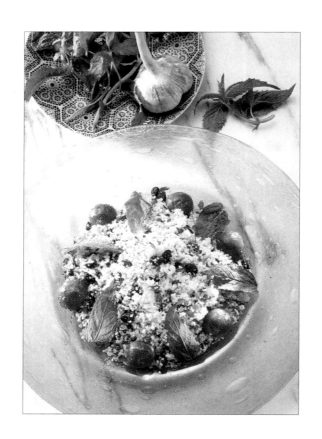

2

Vegetarian

O ver the past few years we have been bombarded by the arguments for and against vegetarianism. Many of us are appalled by the rough treatment some animals receive at the hands of some farmers. With today's factory farming and high-tech agrochemical methods of rearing animals, the meat in supermarkets and butchers' shops may also contain traces of chemicals and antibiotics. As meat is further up the food chain than plant matter, substances such as pesticides and fertilisers that are used to farm vegetable crops may occur in the animals that feed on these crops. This explains why people are increasingly buying organic meat, cutting down on the amount of meat they eat, or more radically, becoming vegetarian.

THE PROTEIN PROBLEM

In general, vegetarians tend to have a healthy diet consisting of plenty of complex carbohydrates (grains, nuts, potatoes, pulses and legumes) and lots of nutritious fruits and vegetables. These healthy vegetarians will be getting all the protein they need from a combination of wholegrains and pulses or from dairy produce and eggs. But those who do not make these foods a regular part of their diet, and many vegetarians opt for the convenience of ready-made meals, may not be getting the intake of protein their bodies require.

Amino acids are the unsung heroes that make up every type of protein in our foods. About twenty different amino acids have been identified so far and, of these, nine cannot be made by the human body. So it is essential that we obtain them from the food we eat. These nine essential amino acids are isoleucine, leucine, lysine, methionine, phenylalanine, threonine, tryptophan, histidine and valine and they each have an important part to play in maintaining a healthy body. Together they are needed for producing haemoglobin (responsible for feeding our cells with oxygen), skin growth, wound healing and to protect the immune system, among other key body processes.

Proteins from animal sources, such as milk and eggs, contain all nine amino acids in approximately the proportions the body needs, and are hence called 'complete' proteins. However, vegetarians should not rely on dairy products and eggs for their entire protein intake but make use of other sources, since dairy foods such as butter and milk are also high in saturated fat. If eaten in excess, saturated fat can cause a build-up of cholesterol in the body and has been linked to serious diseases.

At this point it is worth mentioning the soya bean. This is a non-animal food that contains all nine essential amino acids, and so soya beans and soya products are particularly important for vegetarians and vegans (who do not eat any dairy produce). It is important to note that other non-animal sources of protein, such as legumes (pulses, beans, nuts and lentils) other than soya beans and common grains, are 'incomplete' proteins. This means that they do not contain all the essential amino acids and they therefore need to be properly combined to provide all the protein we need. To make complete protein from incomplete proteins, eat:

- ☐ Legumes with grains/nuts and seeds, e.g. beans on toast
- ☐ Grains with legumes, e.g. nut risotto
- ☐ Nuts and seeds with legumes, e.g. peanut butter and sesame seed sandwich

Glorious Grains

Grains have been the staple diet of many civilisations for thousands of years: wheat, oats, barley and rye in Europe; Maize (or sweetcorn) in America; rice in the East and millet in Africa. In their natural, unrefined state, i.e. bread made from wholemeal flour and brown rice, grains are highly

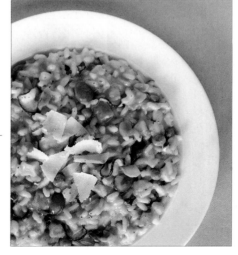

nutritious and are an important source of protein and minerals.

Legumes

There are several thousand varieties of beans and peas which all belong to the legume family. Legumes are unusual vegetables as they contain 17–25 percent protein, roughly double that of wholegrains. They also contain useful amounts of iron, potassium, calcium, vitamin C and niacin (vitamin B3). As we have seen soya beans are a particularly important source of protein for vegetarians and there are numerous soya products available including soya milk and tofu – which can be added to soups and sauces. Other popular beans are aduki, black-eyed, borlotti, kidney, butter, flageolet, haricot, broad and runner beans – so there is a bean to suit every palate.

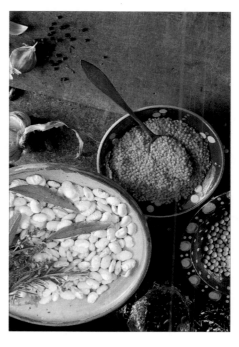

There are also several varieties of peas. Chick-peas are particularly popular and their savoury flavour gives humus its distinctive taste. Dried peas, often called blue peas, are tasty and excellent in stews and soups. Split peas, available in yellow or green, make a good purée for serving with vegetables.

Lentils also come in different colours and are a good source of protein and rich in iron. They are frequently used in Indian cooking and form the basis of dhal. Use green lentils in curries or to thicken soups and sauces.

Sprouted beans and pulses

Many beans, pulses and seeds, such as alfalfa, can be successfully sprouted. This can easily be done at home, simply by leaving the beans or grains on a clean, damp tea cloth on the window-sill or in an airing cupboard. Sprouting increases the vitamin, mineral and enzyme levels of beans, pulses and seeds dramatically. The most successful varieties of pulses for sprouting are alfalfa, lentils and mung beans. When sprouted,

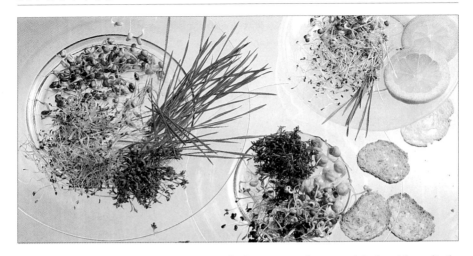

they are delicious eaten raw in salads or simply sprinkled with a little freshly squeezed lemon juice. Alfalfa sprouts are particularly important for vegetarians as they are a 'complete' protein and also contain calcium, B vitamins (including B12) and several enzymes to improve digestion. They can be bought as seeds and sprouted before eating to release their valuable nutrients.

Seeds

Despite their size, seeds are packed with vitamins, minerals and protein and they make a tasty snack or a rich addition to many recipes. Pumpkin seeds contain useful amounts of calcium, zinc and iron as well as some B vitamins. Sesame seeds are an excellent source of calcium and protein as are sunflower seeds. Sunflower seeds are also rich in essential fatty acids that help to keep our cholesterol levels in check.

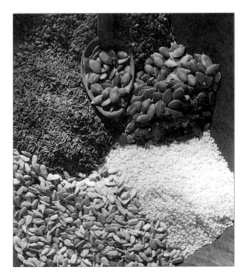

Nuts

Nuts are rich in vitamin E and many minerals including zinc, potassium and calcium. All nuts should be eaten raw and as fresh

as possible as they turn rancid when exposed to heat and light. For this reason it is best to avoid processed or dry-roasted nuts, which are also highly salted. Nuts last longest when stored in an airtight container in the fridge. There are so many to choose from: almonds, brazils, cashews, hazelnuts, chestnuts, coconut and walnuts. Not only are they great to snack on, they can also be added to stir-fries, rice dishes and salads. One of the most popular nuts, the peanut, is not really a nut at all. It belongs to the same legume family as the soya bean and is especially rich in protein, iron, vitamin E and B vitamins (including folic acid).

Caution: Some people suffer a serious allergic reaction after eating nuts. Please consult your doctor if you are in any doubt.

Fruit and vegetables

Last, but definitely not least, a vegetarian diet should contain an abundance of fresh fruit and vegetables. There are hundreds of varieties to choose from – all packed with vitamins, minerals and enzymes. The majority of fruits and vegetables contain very little fat, if any, and this is usually of the healthy polyunsaturated kind.

To get the best from fruit and vegetables, it is advisable to buy organic. It is an undisputed fact of farming life that modern methods of cultivation have contaminated our soil, crops and water supplies with pesticides and chemical fertilisers. These chemicals work by supplying the soil with the basic ingredients for plant growth: nitrogen (in the form of nitrates), phosphorus, potassium and calcium. Unfortunately, by overloading the earth with these elements the delicate balance of other vitally important trace elements, such as magnesium, is disrupted. By contrast, organic farmers tend to use more environmentally friendly fertilisers that include manure, seaweed, herbs such as comfrey, and mineral-enriched rock dust to feed the soil with a complete spectrum of nutrients. Crops grown the organic way end up with a higher nutritional content and contain extra protein, more vitamin C and minerals such as calcium and iron. They are also free from chemical pesticides and are not sprayed with toxic fungicides.

Other fruit and vegetables are sprayed with numerous chemicals to protect them against fungi and insect infestation. This may produce good-looking produce, but it could be to the detriment of our health. The toxic chemicals are absorbed into the skins of fruit and vegetables and eventually end up in our bodies when we eat them. The Government now recommend that carrots are peeled before they are eaten and not just scrubbed as recent tests have shown that some poisonous chemicals can be absorbed into the carrot and can only be removed by peeling off the

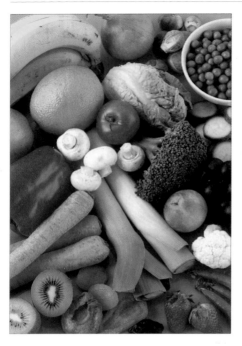

outer layer. It is important to scrub all fruit and vegetables in warm soapy water to remove some of the chemicals, dirt and bacteria that may be present.

If you have trouble finding an organic source, then the Soil Association can provide a list of organic farmers and suppliers in your area (see Useful Addresses). However, it is not always possible to get hold of organic produce, and the next best thing is to buy locally grown produce. If you can't avoid possible residues of synthetic chemicals, at least you can ensure that the nutrient content hasn't been depleted by early harvesting or lengthy storage. The longer a fruit or vegetable is transported or stored, the less nutrients it contains. Produce from abroad is often picked well before it ripens which means it has less time to gather essential nutrients from the soil. Buying locally grown fruit and vegetables in season helps us to keep in touch with the ebb and flow of nature's cycle and ensures we get the nutrients we need when we need them. Don't be afraid to ask your supplier or local supermarket where their produce comes from. Local greengrocers normally have a good idea of where their fruit and vegetables are grown and they might even be persuaded to stock organic produce. Alternatively, to guarantee that your fruit and vegetables are organic, tasty and nutritious, you can try growing your own.

IMPORTANT VITAMINS AND MINERALS FOR VEGETARIANS

Vegetarians may find it difficult to get some key vitamins and minerals from their diet. Those that are listed on pages 33–5 are mainly found in animal foods, so vegetarians may consider taking a supplement to ensure that their bodies are not lacking these nutrients.

Warning: Children's nutritional requirements differ from those of adults.

Iron plays a vital role in the production of red blood cells which carry oxygen from our lungs to all body cells in order to give us energy. It also helps the body to fight infection. Iron deficiency is fairly common in women and this often causes anaemia, insufficient production of red blood cells. Symptoms of anaemia are tiredness, fatigue and lack of stamina. It has been estimated that in the western world 30 percent of women of child-bearing age and about the same percentage of children are lacking iron. Good vegetarian sources of iron are dried apricots, figs, spinach, broccoli, fortified breakfast cereals and wholemeal bread as well as other less well-known grains. Cereals supply 45 percent of the iron intake for non-vegetarians, but almost 100 percent for vegetarians. This form of iron is more difficult for the body to absorb than iron from animal sources. Fortunately vitamin C aids iron absorption in the body, so try to eat vitamin C-rich foods at the same time as eating foods with a high iron content. For example, add some freshly chopped strawberries to a bowl of bran flakes for breakfast with a glass of fresh orange juice and eat an orange or a kiwi fruit after a spinach flan or brown rice risotto (both of which are rich in iron). Alternatively, consider taking iron and vitamin C supplements, but make sure that you follow the instructions carefully when taking iron supplements as too much iron can be harmful. A very high consumption of fibre can interfere with the absorption of iron, as can high tannin intakes, such as from tea.

Vitamin B2 (riboflavin) is involved in energy metabolism and the development of healthy skin, hair and nails. Its best vegetarian sources are milk, eggs, fortified bread and breakfast cereals, green leafy vegetables and yeast extract. Some vegetarians, particularly those who do not eat dairy produce, may find it difficult to meet their daily requirements of this vitamin and may lack energy as a result.

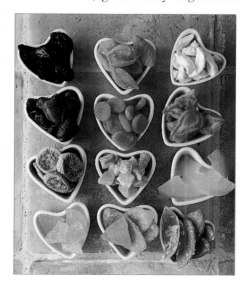

Vitamin B12 is essential for the formation of red blood cells. It is involved in maintaining a healthy nervous system and in energy production. Although it is important to have a daily intake of B12, the body stores this vitamin in the liver. Therefore, if your diet is lacking vitamin B12 on a certain day, your body can use its stores to make up the balance.

Unfortunately for vegetarians, vitamin B12 is mostly found naturally in foods of animal origin such as offal, meat, poultry, fish, eggs and dairy produce, although sprouted alfalfa seeds and Marmite are good sources. Fortunately, many breakfast cereals are fortified with B vitamins. Those who find it difficult to maintain their energy levels may be lacking vitamin B12 and may be required to take a B12 supplement. Smokers and alcohol drinkers may also require a daily dose.

Zinc is essential for normal growth and development. It is also required for the production and maintenance of proteins and so it affects our rate of growth. In addition, zinc aids the development of the

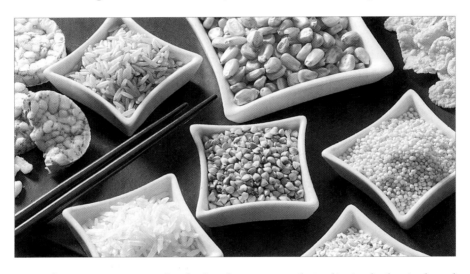

reproductive organs, and a lack of it can result in limited physical and sexual development. We also need zinc to form healthy teeth and bones and to maintain the immune system. It even helps wounds to heal quickly. The best sources of zinc are foods of animal origin as their protein content helps the body to absorb this important trace element. As a result, there is concern that vegetarians and vegans may require an increased zinc intake. Good non-animal sources of zinc are carrots, roasted peanuts, canned tomatoes, peas, sweetcorn and wholemeal bread. However, a high intake of fibre and excessive intakes of alcohol, iron and calcium can all interfere with its absorption.

Calcium is an essential mineral for both children and adults as it is needed for the development and maintenance of strong bones and teeth. It also plays an important role in normal blood clotting as well as regulating our heartbeat. As we get older, our bodies begin to lose calcium and we find it more difficult to absorb. It is thought that a reduction of the level of vitamin D is partly to blame for this, as this vitamin is essential for the absorption of calcium from food (as we age, we tend to spend less time outdoors in the sunlight, which is our main source of vitamin D). Dairy products are good sources of calcium, so vegans will find it hard to meet their bodies' calcium requirements. Fortunately, green leafy vegetables such as broccoli are good sources, as are peanuts, although it may be simpler for some vegetarians and vegans to take a calcium supplement.

Vitamin D is produced by the body under the skin as a result of exposure to the sun's UV rays, which is why it is often referred to as the 'sunshine vitamin'. Its main function in the body is to aid absorption of calcium and phosphorus to form healthy teeth and bones. However, you do not need to sit in the sun for long periods in order for your body to manufacture enough vitamin D. Over-exposure to the sun's ultra-violet rays can cause the skin to burn.

Iodine is difficult for meat eaters and vegetarians alike to obtain from their daily diet. It is naturally present in soil and the levels of iodine in meat, vegetables and cereals alike depend upon the amount of iodine present in the soil on which these grains and animals feed. Unfortunately, the level of iodine in soil varies considerably around the world, so we cannot always rely on these foods to supply enough of the mineral. We need iodine for regulating the thyroid gland and controlling our metabolism, which is important if we are to maintain a steady weight and get the energy we need from our diet. Seafoods are our richest source of iodine, so vegans and vegetarians who do not eat fish are more likely to be missing out on this important nutrient. Sea vegetables such as seaweeds are a rich source for vegetarians or vegans. Alternatively, to ensure that you are getting enough iodine there are plenty of supplements available – kelp supplements are particularly rich in iodine.

For more information about being a healthy vegetarian and over forty recipes, see my *Quick Guide to Vegetarian Cookery* (Boxtree).

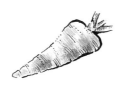

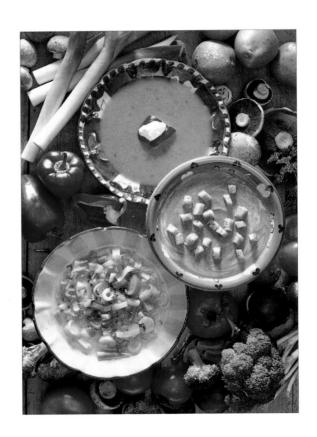

CHAPTER 3

Dieting

Around 20 percent of all women and as many as 25 percent of teenagers go on a diet *each year* in the hope of attaining a slender figure. With the waif-like forms of supermodels as role models for modern women, the pressure to be slim has never been greater. Some women are on diets throughout their lives and cannot eat anything without feeling guilty. Those on highly restricted diets are often cutting important foods from their diet and depriving their body of certain nutrients. In the Sixties and Seventies some of the worst fad diets encouraged women to eat nothing but eggs and grapefruit or bananas and milk. Today we are far more aware of the importance of nutrition and that these severely restricted diets are bad for our overall well-being.

WHY MOST DIETS DON'T WORK

According to the Government's 1992 *Dietary and Nutritional Survey of British Adults*, around one-fifth of the population is following a rigid dieting regime at any one moment in time. The average length of these diets is six and a half weeks for women and ten weeks for men. So why aren't all these diets working? The plain, unpalatable truth is that short-term, fad diets simply don't lead to long-term weight-loss. In fact, they are more likely to cause more harm than good. This is because short-term dieting triggers the damaging Yo-Yo effect. For example, if you start a fad diet that only allows you to eat a few hundred calories a day, the body believes it is at risk of starvation and quickly responds by conserving energy. This leads to a lowering of our basic metabolic rate, which controls how quickly we burn our food as fuel.

The problem with lowering our metabolism is that the body adapts and learns to survive on fewer calories. Scientists have recognised that once the metabolism has been lowered by frugal eating, it is hard to boost it back to its previous level when the diet is stopped. During a period of intense food restriction you might only be eating around 1,000 calories a day, so the body becomes adept at functioning on this low calorific intake. This means that when you return to your previous calorie intake of around 2,000 calories a day, the body may store the extra calories in the form of fat. Not only will your original weight-loss quickly return, but you are likely to end up feeling constantly hungry and so pile on the pounds more easily than before. This rebound at the end of a period of dieting is one of the key reasons why so many diets don't work in the long term.

The long-term risk factors of crash dieting followed by weight gain may also dangerously increase the risk of heart disease and strokes. The healthiest way to lose those excess pounds is to follow a steady long-term weight-loss programme full of wholesome, natural foods that are high in fibre and low in fat and sugar, whilst speeding up your metabolism with regular exercise.

The Healthy Eating Guidelines set out in the Busy chapter of this book form the basis for healthy, long-term weight-loss. Simply cut down on processed foods, such as ready-made meals, and stock your cupboards with a mixture of wholegrains, fruits, vegetables, legumes, nuts and seeds. These vitality foods are, pound for pound, more nutritious and less fattening than manufactured products. Natural foods, such as wholegrains – wheat, brown rice, fruits and vegetables – are also high in fibre, whereas most processed foods are stripped of their fibre content. All nutritionists agree that one of the most important rules of any healthy weight-loss plan is to eat much more in the way of carbohydrates – rice, bread, pasta – because they are packed with fibre. High-fibre foods make us feel full on fewer calories and also tend to be low in fat and sugar. To satisfy hunger pangs between meals, snack on fruits and vegetables which are low in calories and rich in fibre, vitamins and minerals.

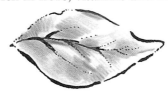

THE FAT FACTOR

A low-fat diet is the number one improvement you can make to achieve weight-loss for life and encourage lasting good health. A healthy diet should contain no more than 35 percent calories from fat, but a weight-loss diet should contain between 20 and 25 percent calories from fat. This will not only help us achieve long-term weight-loss, it will also dramatically reduce our risk of cancer and heart disease. Population studies all over the world reveal a close link between a diet high in saturated fat and an increased risk of heart disease and certain types of cancer. One of the easiest ways to monitor the amount of fat we eat each day is to keep track of our fat grams. This method of weight watching is especially popular in America, where it has largely replaced calorie counting.

FAT GRAM FINDERS

HIGH FAT		LOW FAT	
Type	Fat grams/portion	Type	Fat grams/portion
Pork pie	30g		
Samosa	26g		
Streaky bacon, fried	25g	Streaky bacon, grilled	20g
Steak and kidney pie	24g		
Sausages	21g	Fat-reduced sausages	11g
Pork chop, grilled	20g		
Small beefburger	20g		
Cheddar cheese	19g	Cottage cheese	2g
Thin-cut chips	17g	Thick-cut chips	8g
Small bar chocolate	15g		
Minced beef	14g	Minced beef, fat poured off	6g
Edam cheese	13g		
Double cream	13g	Single cream	6g
Small bag of peanuts	12g		
Roast chicken, with skin	12g	Roast chicken, without skin	4g
Fish fingers, fried	11g	Fish fingers, grilled	6g
Halva	11g		
Small bag of crisps	11g	Fat-reduced crisps	7g
Butter or margarine	8g		
Roast potatoes	8g	Boiled or baked potatoes	0g

SUGAR SENSE

We are a nation of sugarholics. Confectionery sales totalling £2,332 million in 1984 were greater than the combined sum spent on bread and cereals. All types of sugar are high in calories and, after fat, are the next most powerful diet-breakers. In addition to piling on the pounds, sugar has been linked to diabetes and skin disorders. As with fat, there are many different ways to describe sugar on food labels. Some may believe that one type of sugar may be better for us than others, but the fact is that sugar, sucrose, glucose, dextrose and all the other 'oses' have no nutritional value other than feeding the body with empty calories.

In fact, having a sugary snack can actually increase our appetite. After eating a sugary snack our blood sugar levels rise dramatically giving us a sudden spurt of energy. However this energy spurt is quickly followed by a more lasting low. This is because insulin is secreted when blood sugar levels are high to bring them quickly back to normal. When our blood sugar levels drop like this we are often left feeling hungrier than before. This is not a true hunger, as we only ate the sweets initially as a quick snack, but it fools the brain into believing that the stomach is empty.

Sugar, therefore, not only rots the teeth, but can also trigger the appetite. If you have a sweet tooth and want to eat sugar, only eat it with a meal so that the rate of absorption is slowed down. If you yearn for a sweet snack, have a piece of fruit instead as the intrinsic sugars in fruits and vegetables are far healthier than the extrinsic sugar present in confectionery and processed foods. Artificial sweeteners may also stimulate the appetite by triggering the release of gastric juices in the stomach in the anticipation of a raised blood glucose level. Hunger pangs may then follow as the sweeteners fail to provide any of the expected calories. For this reason it is also best to use chemical sweeteners at meal times. If you drink a beverage with artificial sweeteners, then try to eat a small snack at the same time, although drinking without eating will not cause you any harm.

THINK SLIM

We should not feel guilty about what we eat or simply blame the foods we enjoy the most for our excess weight. If your favourite food is cheese, which has a very high fat content, then you should not feel the need to cut it out of your diet completely – merely limit the amount of cheese you eat each week. If you give up all the foods you enjoy the most, then you are more likely to become fed up with your diet and seek solace in fattening comfort foods. Food is our life-source and we must not think of it as our enemy. Instead, make friends with food and experiment with different fruits, vegetables, grains, herbs and spices to create really delicious, low-fat meals. Diets do not have to be boring and with the abundance of luscious fresh produce, interesting grains and tasty herbs available all year round, your meals need not lack variety.

SUPPLEMENTS FOR LOW-FAT DIETS

Whatever diet you are on, it is vitally important to make sure that you are getting your daily requirements of all the vitamins and minerals your body needs. Those who are on low-fat diets will probably be cutting down on dairy products because of their high-fat content. However, butter,

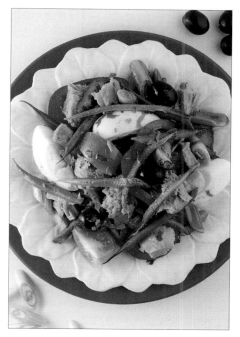

cheese, cream, milk and yoghurt are important sources of calcium, vitamin A, vitamin D and biotin (a B vitamin), so look out for low-fat alternatives of these foods. We need calcium and vitamin D to maintain healthy teeth and bones, vitamin A for everyday bodily functions and biotin for energy and to maintain healthy skin, hair and bone marrow. Fortunately if you eat plenty of fruit and vegetables every day, your body will create all the vitamin A it needs from the beta-carotene present in these foods. Other good sources of calcium are green leafy vegetables, and vitamin D can be found in cod liver oil, kippers, mackerel, canned salmon and eggs. Biotin is found in wholemeal bread and brown rice. However, if you do not eat any of the above foods regularly, consider supplementing your diet with these nutrients.

Other high-fat foods include nuts, seeds, avocados and vegetable oils such as olive oil, which are 100 percent fat! However, these fats are polyunsaturated and far healthier than the saturated fat found in meat and dairy produce. Vegetable oils, such as olive oil and grapeseed oil, contain important nutrients that we miss out on if we cut all fat from our diet. They are rich sources of essential fatty acids which the body cannot produce itself, so they must be obtained from our diet. Essential fatty acids maintain healthy cell membranes and form prostaglandins, which control a number of processes within the body. Some fish, such as cod, mackerel and herring, are also rich in essential fatty acids, but if you don't eat much fish, it is worth taking a cod liver oil supplement.

Another vitamin that slimmers often lack is vitamin E as this is found mainly in vegetable oils and nuts which are high in fat. Vitamin E is an important antioxidant that protects fatty tissues and cells. It is also found in wheatgerm, eggs, wholemeal bread and green leafy vegetables.

ENERGY-BOOSTING SUPPLEMENTS

One of the problems of many diets is the lack of energy slimmers often feel due to their restricted calorie intake. Fortunately, there are numerous nutrients which can help us to create energy more effectively from our reduced intake of food. The B-complex vitamins, made up of B1 (thiamine), B2 (riboflavin), B5 (pantothenic acid), B6 (pyridoxine), B9 (folic acid) and B12 (cobalamin), together form a powerful energy-boosting supplement. They work synergistically to release energy from the food we eat. The mineral magnesium is also needed to convert the food we eat into energy as well as being an essential part of our bones. Foods rich in magnesium include soya beans, nuts, wholemeal bread, pasta, peas, seafood, green vegetables and dried fruit.

Iron gives us energy in a different way. It plays a vital role in the production of red blood cells which carry oxygen from our lungs to all body cells. Our cells need oxygen to use food as a source of energy. The richest sources of iron are offal and red meat. Vitamin C aids iron absorption from foods and also helps to boost the body's defences against infection which may be at a low ebb during a restricted diet. Vitamin C is mainly found in kiwi fruit, blackcurrants, strawberries and green vegetables. Zinc also helps to boost our immune reactions and its best sources are seafood, red meat, dairy produce and some green vegetables and cereals.

EXERCISE

A reduced calorie diet that is high in fibre and low in fat will enable you to lose weight healthily in the long term, but exercise is needed to tone your body and create a trimmer, firmer figure. Exercise also enables us to burn calories more effectively and will therefore aid weight-loss (see the Calorie Counter). Aerobic exercise is best as it not only burns up excess fat and calories, but also greatly improves the performance of our heart and lungs. Aerobic exercise does not refer to aerobic classes alone, although this is a sure and fast way to burn up those excess calories. Other forms of aerobic exercise include cycling, jogging, swimming or even just

walking. In order to maximise the benefits of exercise, you need to aim to exercise for twenty minutes or more at least three times a week.
Caution: If you suffer from a medical condition, consult your doctor before undertaking a new exercise regime.

JOIN A GYM

If there are particular areas of your body that need to be toned then it may be worthwhile joining a gym. Modern gyms are equipped with different machines to target every major muscle in the body – even those muscles that are hard to exercise, such as the inner thigh. Many of the council-run leisure centres have gyms that are far cheaper to join than privately run sports clubs, and they often have reduced prices for students and the unemployed. So investigate your local leisure centre and see what facilities are available.

CALORIE COUNTER

EXERCISE	Approx. Kcals per hour	EXERCISE	Approx. Kcals per hour
Step aerobics	600	Tennis	450
Skipping	600	Cycling	400
Aerobics	550	Badminton	350
Swimming	500	Fast walking	300

WHICH EXERCISE?

Choose from the list below to find out which form of aerobic exercise is best suited to you and your lifestyle.

Aerobics: It is best to choose low-impact aerobics rather than the high-impact variety as this is more gentle on your joints, especially if you have not done aerobics before. Almost every health club or sports centre runs aerobic classes and the fact that everything is organised for you is more incentive to go on a regular basis. There are also numerous aerobic workout videos available which you can follow in the comfort of your own home. Before you embark on any aerobic exercise it is vitally important that you carry out stretching and warming up exercises first, as these prepare your body for what is in store. If you are suffering from any medical condition which may be affected by exercising, such as a back problem, then you should consult your doctor first.
Cycling: This is an excellent form of aerobic exercise which is not tough on your joints, and it will greatly tone your legs. Cycling is also a great

form of transport, but not when it is done on busy main roads where not only do you have to stop and start all the time, but you are also breathing in fumes from cars and diesel lorries. Today, of course, you can cycle in the comfort of your own home on static exercise bikes.

Dancing: Exercise does not have to be a repetitive routine of the same short movements, it can also be in the form of something creative such as dance. Dancing, whether it be disco dancing or ballet, may be something which you enjoy doing already for its own sake. So if you have a busy night life, it is no excuse for not doing any exercise, as the dance floor is the ideal place for some serious blood pumping.

Jogging and running: These two types of exercise really get the blood surging! But they are not suitable for those who have problems with their weight-bearing joints, such as knees or ankles. You should avoid running or jogging on concrete pavements or other hard ground as this puts even greater pressure on your joints. Make sure you wear proper running shoes which provide adequate support and cushioning. If there is a field or park near you then use this, as grass has a certain amount of 'give' which is ideal for this type of aerobic exercise.

Walking: Even this everyday activity is aerobic if you put enough energy into it. Either on your way to work or in your lunch hour, you should spend at least ten solid minutes each day walking briskly. To get the best from walking, your back should be straight, tummy in, and as you walk sway your hips subtly to either side while swinging your arms. Walking this way not only encourages excellent posture, it also exercises your

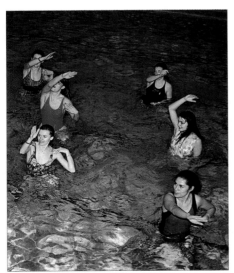

bottom, thighs and arms. The more movement involved in your walk, the more aerobic it is and the more calories you will burn. As with all other exercises, it is best if you walk in fresh air to ensure that you inhale large amounts of oxygen and few fumes.

Rebounding: Rebounding on a mini trampoline (or bouncer) is another great form of aerobic exercise and it is believed by some to be the best possible form of exercise for combating cellulite due to the use it makes of the force of gravity. The up-and-

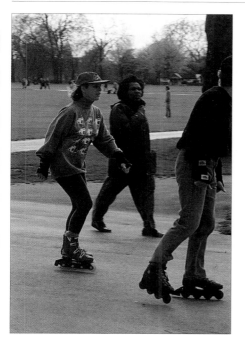

down movement, which first suspends your body in space and then subjects it to two or three times the force of gravity, stimulates the elimination of wastes through your lymphatic system. Increased oxygen is also brought to the cells, boosting the whole system and encouraging general detoxification. Rebounding is something that you can do in the privacy of your own home irrespective of your age, your level of fitness or the weather outside. You can bounce to music or in front of the television and you can even skip at the same time. Another benefit is that you will never be troubled by constipation if you rebound regularly.

Rollerblading / skating: This exhilarating sport is not only a fun way to get around, it is also great exercise for the muscles in your calves, thighs and buttocks. Rollerblading should be performed on smooth, dry surfaces, well away from busy roads. Parks are ideal, but consideration must be shown for pedestrians, cyclists and other park users. Once you have mastered the technique of rollerblading and skating, it is possible to reach speeds of up to 30 miles per hour, so always be aware of possible obstructions. A helmet and protective clothing should be worn.

Swimming: This is a great exercise for toning your whole body and it does not have the problems which weight-bearing exercises have. Even those who have weak ankles, knees or backs can swim, as your body becomes weightless in water and so removes any pressure on these areas. When swimming, you are exercising virtually every major muscle in your body but the water keeps you cool. To get the best out of swimming, you need to swim straight lengths without stopping to rest, for at least twenty minutes. If this is your only exercise, try and do it three times a week, every other day. You could also slip in a few underwater hip- and thigh-toning exercises at the end of your swimming session. Any exercise you do underwater involves a great deal more effort than on land as the weight of the water restricts your movements.

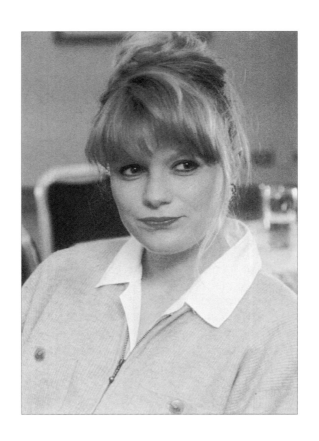

4

Monthly cycle

An estimated 10 million women in Britain suffer from premenstrual syndrome, or PMS, a collection of physical and mental symptoms that begin anything between two and fourteen days before menstruation. The actual symptoms, which include depression, stomach cramps and breast pains, vary widely from woman to woman. Some women may just feel a little discomfort each month, while others may experience devastating psychological effects. There have been several cases of unusually violent behaviour in women linked to PMS. Nicola Owen made legal history when she was the first woman successfully to use PMS as a mitigating plea in the courts. She was discharged from the Old Bailey where she had faced charges of arson after trying to commit suicide by setting fire to the family home. Eighteen-year-old Anna Reynolds killed her mother with a hammer but was released from a life sentence on appeal after two years on the strength of medical evidence of the severity of her premenstrual symptoms. Both women's PMS later responded positively to hormone and dietary treatment.

WHAT ARE THE SYMPTOMS?

All of the symptoms in the following table have been reported by women premenstrually. If you experience any of these symptoms each month then they are probably related to PMS. For different women, the type and severity of symptoms vary widely. There may also be changes over time, for example, after having children the monthly symptoms may become more severe.

SYMPTOMS OF PMS

PSYCHOLOGICAL	PHYSICAL
Altered sex drive	Abdominal bloating and discomfort
Anger and aggression	Acne
Anxiety and panic attacks	Asthma
Change in sexual desire	Backache
Clumsiness	Breast swelling or tenderness
Crying uncontrollably, often for no apparent reason	Cold sore recurrence, if already infected
Depression	Dizziness
Feelings of insecurity	Fainting
Hunger and food cravings, especially for sugary foods	Fatigue and loss of energy
Irritability	Headaches and migraine
Loss of control	Joint pains
Low self-worth	Lower back pain
Mood swings	Nausea or vomiting
Phobias	Palpitations
Suicidal feelings	Rashes
Tension	Runny nose
	Sinusitis
	Sore eyes or throat
	Swollen legs or ankles
	Visual disturbances
	Weight gain

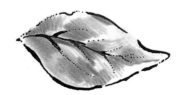

COMMON SYMPTOMS

MOOD CHANGES

Many women say they feel a different person before their period. They can become intensely irritable and snappy with everyone – husband, kids, workmates, even the doctor, or worse, the boss. The forgetfulness and inability to focus attention that often accompanies this makes even the simplest tasks take much longer than they should – increasing the sense of frustration. At other times the mood is one of deep depression, and self-confidence flies out of the window. Some women also experience attacks of irrational panic or anxiety and seem to have no control over their emotions.

TENDER BREASTS

It is quite common for breasts to enlarge in the two weeks before a period, returning to normal after the period begins. Premenstrual breast pain affects some five million women in Britain between the ages of twenty and fifty. It can affect part or all of the breast and even extend to the upper arms. Other breast problems include nodularity or lumpiness in the breast just before a period.

ABDOMINAL DISTENSION, WEIGHT GAIN

One of the most commonly reported symptoms of PMS is weight gain, and it can also be one of the most upsetting. Many women regularly report putting on several pounds overnight, waking up with a puffy face, swollen ankles and an uncomfortable, bloated abdomen. In fact the weight gain is just water retention, and it will almost certainly disappear as quickly as it came shortly after the period starts.

CLUMSINESS

Dropping things, forgetfulness, confusion. This is particularly distressing if you are in a job where you have to keep your mind sharp, because such symptoms can be mistaken for inability and incompetence. If you also suffer from tension premenstrually (PMT), then accidentally dropping a plate, banging your head or losing your car keys can be guaranteed to take you to screaming point.

HEADACHES, SUGAR CRAVINGS, LETHARGY

These can all result from erratic swings in blood sugar levels. Snacking on sugary sweets or overdosing on caffeine can not only contribute to the cause, it can make matters worse. A sweet snack might boost energy levels temporarily, but it will soon be followed by fatigue. You respond to that with another, similar snack... and you could find yourself on a roller-coaster of activity and lethargy. Dietary strategies are particularly effective with these symptoms, and will be discussed later.

WHAT CAUSES PMS?

There have been several thousand research papers on the subject of PMS and, although doctors are more aware of the different ways in which the symptoms can be treated, we are still a long way from understanding why exactly PMS happens. However, the fact that both oestrogen and progesterone are produced in huge quantities around the time that we experience PMS means they seem to be the primary culprits. It has been demonstrated that when the ovaries are either removed surgically or have their action suppressed by drugs – so removing the cyclical hormonal changes – the symptoms of PMS usually disappear.

As well as controlling the physical changes that happen to a woman's body during the menstrual cycle, oestrogen and progesterone can also have an effect on mood. Oestrogen can act as a stimulant, resulting in anxiety, irritability and tension, while low levels cause depression. Progesterone, on the other hand, is a depressant. So a correct balance between the two hormones throughout the cycle is important. Too much prolactin from the pituitary gland can upset the balance between these two hormones, resulting in too little progesterone, or too much oestrogen, being produced.

However, it is not just an imbalance of hormones that is to blame for the symptoms of PMS, or we would all experience the same symptoms to the same degree. Experts now believe that the symptoms are caused by the way the body handles the normal fluctuations in our hormone levels, rather than the hormone imbalance itself. So the fault lies in the way we react to our own natural sex hormones. There is also evidence that external factors like stress and diet affect the severity of PMS symptoms. Here are the most common influences on PMS:

Poor diet: In particular, eating too much sugar and saturated fat. Indulging cravings for sweet, sugary foods can cause wild fluctuations in blood sugar levels, which can make us feel in turn shaky then tired, irritable then depressed.

Caffeine: Chinese scientists found that there is a strong association between increased caffeine consumption and severity of premenstrual symptoms. Those women suffering most were also drinking the most coffee. Oestrogen may be to blame as it slows down the rate at which caffeine is broken down by the liver.

Essential fatty acid deficiency: These are the raw materials from which hormones are made. If we are deficient in certain essential fatty acids, hormone production can be affected.

Obesity: Excess fatty tissue has an effect on oestrogen production and so can affect the hormonal balance and increase the symptoms of PMS.

Drugs, alcohol and smoking: Anything that has an effect on mood can in turn exacerbate the mood changes of PMS.

Pollution from petrol fumes, chemical sprays, etc.: Many kinds of pollution can have an effect upon the availability of essential trace elements such as magnesium and zinc, which in turn can influence hormone production.

Oral contraceptives: These and other artificial sources of hormones can influence the body's hormone balance.

Stress: Severe physical or mental stress can actually cause the pituitary gland to bring the monthly action of the ovaries to a complete halt. For example, it is not unusual for professional female athletes to stop having periods altogether through the effect of regular high-level exercise on their hormones. For the rest of us great emotional stress can cause our period to be late or missed altogether.

Pregnancy: Although the nine months of pregnancy usually render a women blissfully free of her regular symptoms, PMS sometimes gets worse afterwards, particularly after a second pregnancy.

Candida albicans, **the yeast infection that causes thrush:** This can either exacerbate or be mistaken for PMS. If you have a tendency to thrush, your PMS symptoms are likely to be worse. Many women develop thrush just before their period.

PMS REMEDIES

EVENING PRIMROSE OIL

Evening primrose oil is known to affect and regulate the action of prostaglandins – hormone-like substances – and has undergone extensive trials to try to pin-point its action in relieving PMS. Several studies have revealed that an important essential fatty acid, gamma-linolenic acid (GLA), present in evening primrose oil is needed to create prostaglandin E1 (PGE1), which controls the balance of our hormones. Essential fatty acids are a small group of compounds found naturally in certain fats, and are vital for health.

Evening primrose oil, like other vegetable oils, also contains linoleic acid which is converted into gamma-linolenic acid and then into PGE1 by means of a series of chemical reactions that take place in the body cells. However, even if you are getting plenty of linoleic acid from your diet in the form of vegetable oils such as sunflower oil, you cannot guarantee you will be able to make all the GLA you need. This is because the enzyme that enables the conversion to take place can only function in the presence of adequate supplies of vitamin B6, zinc and magnesium, so these must also be supplied by the diet. In addition, the enzyme is inhibited by stress, advancing age, virus infections, alcohol consumption and a diet high in sugar and saturated fat. Fortunately, evening primrose oil is a rich source of gamma-linolenic acid and can, therefore, bypass this part of the conversion process and provide the body directly with the GLA it needs to produce PGE1.

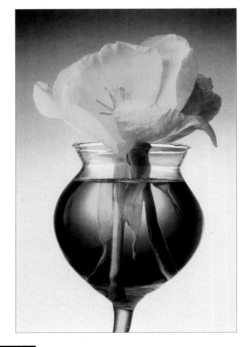

Once gamma-linolenic acid is formed in the body (or supplied from supplements such as evening primrose oil) the next step is for it to be modified into a form called dihomo gamma-linolenic acid (DGLA), and then into PGE1. This final part of the conversion process requires vitamins B3 and C. If the process is blocked at any stage, not enough PGE1 is produced and one of the results is increased sensitivity to prolactin. This heightened sensitivity will affect the production of the sex hormones oestrogen and progesterone, upsetting the balance between the two and causing PMS symptoms.

There have been numerous successful clinical trials demonstrating the positive effect of evening primrose oil in treating PMS symptoms. Premenstrual breast tenderness responds particularly well to treatment with evening primrose oil and patients suffering from mastalgia – severe breast pain – can now obtain the oil on prescription. Evening primrose oil is one of the few natural products to receive a medical licence and many medics believe that it should be the first line of treatment for breast pain.

A GUIDE TO DOSAGE Not everyone requires the same dose of evening primrose to treat their PMS symptoms. The best dose for the individual may be found by a simple process of trial and error to see what works. Evening primrose oil has very few side-effects, even when taken in large doses, so it is fine to experiment with the dosage. The Evening Primrose Office recommends taking 2 x 500mg capsules a day for severe PMS and 2 x 250mg capsules for mild PMS. In most cases, evening primrose oil takes a couple of months before any improvement in severe disorders such as mastalgia is noticed.

Caution: Evening primrose oil should not be taken by anyone with temporal lobe epilepsy. Please note that very large doses may cause stomach upsets.

VITAMIN B6

This vital nutrient is believed to influence hormonal activity by helping the body make more efficient use of available essential fatty acids (see page 13), thus reducing the severity of symptoms. The recommended daily allowance (RDA) of vitamin B6 is 2mg per day, and most people get enough from meat, fish, cereals and vegetables. However, some women do not absorb vitamin B6 from their food effectively. Fortunately, vitamin B6 supplements in quantities of 100–200mg per day can be taken throughout the cycle and can alleviate symptoms of PMS in some women. Again, it may take three months before the benefits of taking B6 start to show, but it's worth persevering. Larger doses taken over long periods of time may cause peripheral neuropathy, symptoms of which include numbness and painful burning sensations in the limbs, which can lead to nerve damage. So if you are planning on buying over-the-counter B6 supplements, seek your GP's advice first on a dose that is likely to be safe and effective for you.

VITAMIN E

This vitamin influences the way we metabolise fats and has been shown to be effective for some symptoms of PMS at doses of between 150mg and 600mg a day. Sufferers of depression and anxiety seem to derive the most benefit. Vitamin E also helps to maintain a healthy blood system. Interestingly, the mineral selenium works synergistically with vitamin E so it is worth taking a supplement combining both nutrients. There are a number of supplements available that combine the two, including those that are sold as antioxidants for their general health benefits. Evening primrose oil capsules also contain vitamin E (as a preservative for the oil).

VITAMIN AND MINERAL SUPPLEMENTS

Modern diets and lifestyle factors may be reducing the amount of minerals that we absorb from our food. For example, magnesium is believed to be lowered by levels of fluoride in the drinking water. Zinc is thought to be lowered by the contraceptive pill, refined carbohydrates (such as white flour and sugar), alcohol, smoking and some food additives. These minerals play an important role in reducing symptoms of PMS, while others, such as iron, are lost during menstruation.

Magnesium: Some, but not all, PMS sufferers have reduced levels of the mineral magnesium in their red blood cells. We don't yet know what part magnesium might play in PMS, although it is needed to convert essential fatty acids into the prostaglandin that balances our hormones. There is some evidence that correcting low magnesium levels relieves symptoms in some women. This is important when you realise that around 15 percent of UK women are probably not getting enough of this essential mineral. Good food sources are nuts, wholegrain cereals, meat and fish.

Zinc: Around one woman in twenty does not get enough zinc in her daily diet. Zinc's roles in the body include hormone production as well as maintaining a healthy immune system and keeping skin healthy. It is found in meat, seafood (especially oysters), yeast and eggs.

Iron: Our levels of this vital mineral can drop dramatically during menstruation so it may be necessary to take an iron supplement. Iron plays a vital role in the production of red blood cells which carry oxygen from our lungs to all body cells to give us energy. It also helps to fight infection. Vitamin C aids the absorption of iron so try to include plenty of vitamin-C rich foods in your meals.

Vitamin B12 and folic acid: These two B vitamins work together to produce red and white blood cells, thus helping to replace those lost in menstruation. They are often included in supplements designed specifically to target PMS.

Calcium: This essential mineral is not ordinarily associated with PMS, but some women who experience menstruation-related migraines have found relief from taking calcium combined with vitamin D. However, too much calcium can deplete our stores of magnesium. Studies have also shown that calcium may help to alleviate other symptoms including water retention and general pain. However, an increased calcium intake may decrease magnesium absorption and magnesium deficiency is linked to PMS.

THE PMS DIET

Although the causes of PMS are many and varied, the severity of the symptoms is to some extent under the individual's control, and diet plays a large part in this. The first principle of a PMS diet is to have a regular intake of complex carbohydrates – bread, pasta, rice, potatoes and other grains and cereals. This helps to normalise blood sugar levels and so reduce the risk of mood swings and food cravings that can occur around this time. Eating frequently throughout the day also helps to keep blood sugar levels in check. Try not to go for more than three hours without a snack, and make sure that all your meals and snacks contain complex carbohydrate foods. Don't worry if you are trying to lose weight as these snacks need not be fattening. A banana or some low-calorie rice cakes is all that is needed to keep your blood sugar levels stable.

Simple sugars are the PMS sufferer's arch enemy. These, for example the granulated sugar you might add to your tea or breakfast cereal, are easily absorbed into the bloodstream where they send our blood glucose levels sky high, until the body over-reacts to compensate and brings them down again so that they are too low. When our blood glucose levels are low, we lack energy and often fall victim to food cravings and this is when PMS symptoms may be triggered.

The saturated fats found in animal fats such as butter, milk and the fat on meats should also not feature too heavily in a PMS diet. Too much saturated fat can in the long term lead to heart disease and may interfere with the absorption of important essential fatty acids that are found in the healthy polyunsaturated fats such as sunflower oil.

The National Association for Premenstrual Syndrome recommend using a chart similar to the one on page 108. Keep a record for three months, or more, before showing your doctor, because it usually takes at least this long to identify a pattern.

For more information, see my *Quick Guide to Beating PMS* (Boxtree)

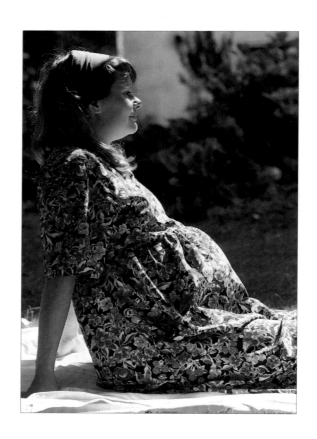

5

Pregnancy

Deciding to have a baby is one of the most creative and exciting choices we can make in life and it's well worth taking several steps towards good healthcare for you and your partner before conception. Although pregnancy isn't like running a marathon, you will find it easier both to get pregnant and to enjoy the nine months with a well-tuned body. Being in good shape will also give your baby the best conditions in which to develop into a healthy human being.

PLANNING FOR PARENTHOOD

Getting pregnant is not always as simple as it sounds. You may conceive the first time you try or it could happen several months later. The average woman takes six months to conceive and may have to wait as long as eighteen months. When planning a baby, it's worth preparing your body from about three to six months before you actually want to conceive. Start to exercise regularly – about three times a week, for twenty minutes each session. Try swimming, jogging, walking, aerobics or playing tennis. This will get your body ready for the load-bearing requirements of pregnancy and the demands of labour. It will also provide a healthy environment in which the foetus can develop. Don't worry if you are already pregnant, now is simply the time to adopt a new healthy diet and lifestyle.

FEMALE FERTILITY

If you have been taking the birth control pill, change to barrier or natural methods of contraception for three months before you want to conceive. This will help your body get back to its normal patterns and prevent any doubts about the time of conception. You may wish to visit your doctor before you conceive – just for a general check-up and for advice on fertility, conception, antenatal care and any other questions you may have on childbirth. It's also worth having a blood test to check that you are immune to German measles (rubella). This illness is mild in adults and children, but can have terrible effects on an unborn child during the first twelve weeks of development. If you aren't immune, you should have a vaccination and avoid conceiving for three months. If you're reading this and are already pregnant, don't worry. The vast majority of pregnancies do result in a healthy baby, and advice on preconceptual care is just another way of ensuring that those eating an unhealthy diet can alter their lifestyles before conception.

MALE FERTILITY

Being prepared about six months before you both want to conceive is not as far-fetched as it sounds. For successful conception, it is as important for the male partner to be in good physical shape as it is for the female, particularly as male sperm take about three months to form in the testes. Sperm problems account for 25–30 percent of infertility cases and there are approximately one million sub-fertile males in the UK.

FOOD FOR THOUGHT

A healthy diet and lifestyle is important (not vital) for you and your partner in the months before conception and during the pregnancy. Focusing on your diet before conception will mean that your bloodstream has the right amount of nutrients needed for the first phase of the baby's growth. Equally, your partner should be eating well to ensure he produces healthy sperm – so maximising your chances of conceiving.

Foresight, the Association for the Promotion of Pre-Conceptual Care, was set up to help protect the health of unborn children by advising on care before conception and to examine the environmental effects on preconceptual health. Again, pregnancies are not always planned and you should not worry about not having prepared beforehand. The Association recommends that both partners follow a wholefood diet for several months before they try to conceive. This diet can be followed throughout your pregnancy and is particularly important during the first three months of your baby's prenatal development, as this is when its limbs, skeleton and major organs are formed.

The Foresight diet advises mothers-to-be to avoid convenience and processed foods and to eat as much fresh produce as possible. Foresight also advises drinking filtered or bottled mineral water and suggests that you and your partner vary your eating habits by choosing and combining from the following four main food groups each day:

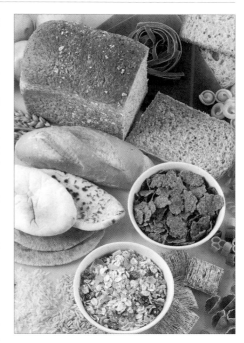

☐ **Cereals:** Eat wholewheat bread, if possible made from organic flour, and wholegrain cereals such as sugar-free muesli. Whole rye, barley, oats, millet, buckwheat, sesame, sunflower seeds and nuts are all good dietary staples. Nuts should be raw and as fresh as possible.

☐ **Dairy products:** These foods are excellent sources of vitamins B2, B12, D and A as well as minerals such as calcium, zinc and magnesium. It's worth choosing the low-fat and semi-skimmed products to avoid a high intake of saturated fats. Soft cheeses and goat and sheep products should be avoided in pregnancy because of the danger of contracting listeria – an infection which can affect the baby and even cause a miscarriage or still-birth. Make sure you cook eggs well because of the danger of contracting salmonella.

☐ **Vegetables, fruits and juices:** Many fruits and vegetables are high in vitamin C, which is needed during pregnancy to help the baby's tissue function. Eat fresh raw fruit and vegetables as often as possible or have your food very lightly cooked, except for potatoes and unsprouted pulses. Have a fresh salad every day using ingredients such as lettuce, white or red cabbage, cress, cauliflower, radish, tomato, celery, watercress, green and red pepper, carrots and button mushrooms. Liven up your salads with sprouted pulses such as alfalfa and mung beans, or different kinds of nuts – such as walnuts or pine kernels.

Over-boiling or frying vegetables can destroy their valuable vitamin and mineral content. Instead, steam your veg in a stainless steel vegetable steamer as this will retain most of the nutrients. Shallow rather than deep-fat frying will also maintain more of the vegetables' goodness.

☐ **Protein foods:** This includes all meat, heart, sweetbreads, tongue, poultry, game and fish, especially shellfish and roe. Protein is needed for the growth and development of new tissue and is essential during pregnancy. Buy your meat as fresh as possible and look for organic and free-range varieties. Foresight also recommends that you consider switching to foods such as venison, rabbit, game-birds, pigeons and all seafoods, as the animals live in their natural environment and are not intensively farmed in the way

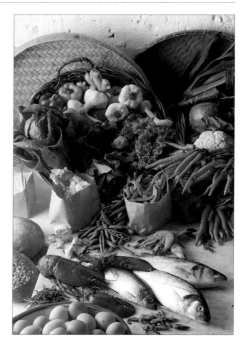

cows and chickens are. Roast or stew your meat with stock or vegetables as the stock will contain much of the meat's valuable nutrients. Large quantities of liver, kidney and pâté should also be avoided as they contain high levels of vitamin A, which may be harmful to the foetus.

WHAT TO AVOID

It's worth cutting all white flour and white flour products (such as white bread, cakes, pasta and white rice) out of your diet. Sweets, jams and fizzy drinks should also be off your menu as these have very little nutritional value. Avoid eating potatoes with green patches as these contain a poisonous alkaloid called solanine, which has been linked to spina bifida in babies. A report by the Government Committee on Toxicology and Carcinogenicity in March 1994 states that there is no conclusive evidence to support this contention and the link remains unproven. However, it is, nonetheless, advisable to avoid green potatoes when pregnant. Try to cut out tinned vegetables, which are usually high in salt and may contain sugar and artificial colouring. Look for salt and sugar-free varieties. Foresight also recommends that mothers-to-be don't eat tinned meat, commercial pâtés, bacon, sausages, or packet ham which often contain preservatives and monosodium glutamate – the latter is usually also present in Chinese take-away food – and which may cause palpitations and faintness.

ESSENTIAL EXTRAS

As well as ensuring you and your partner are eating well, there are various supplements each partner can take to promote a healthy pregnancy. Pregnant women in particular should increase their intake of many nutrients vital for healthy growth and development of the foetus.

FOLIC ACID

This is the most important vitamin supplement a woman can take before and during the first twelve weeks of her pregnancy. It is essential for the proper development of the baby's spine, which takes place in the first four weeks of pregnancy. If the spinal vertebrae do not fuse properly, the baby can be born with spina bifida, which affects nearly 2,000 pregnancies each year. Folic acid is found in green vegetables and fortified cereals, but a pregnant woman's diet usually only contains one-third of the amount needed to prevent a baby's handicap. The Government has recommended that women take a supplement containing 400mcg of the vitamin a day – before and up to the twelfth week of their pregnancy. But remember, starting to take the supplement only later on in pregnancy is too late to protect the unborn child. This is because the neural tubes will have already closed over.

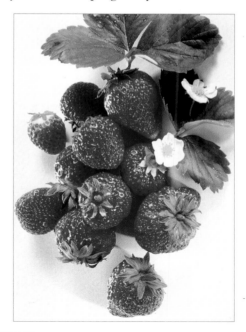

CALCIUM

You need about twice as much calcium as normal during pregnancy. As your baby's bones begin to develop very early in pregnancy, your calcium intake during the first four months is important. It's found in cheese, milk, yoghurt, leafy green vegetables, wholegrains, pulses and nuts.

VITAMIN C

Very important as it helps to build a strong placenta, helps your body fight infection and promotes iron absorption. It is found in fresh fruit and vegetables, such as oranges, grapefruit, strawberries, broccoli, potatoes and cabbage.

IRON

Your body will need a good supply of iron during pregnancy as iron is a vital ingredient of haemoglobin, the substance that carries oxygen to your baby via the bloodstream. Around one-third of your iron intake is used by the baby to create blood and build up its own stores. Found in red meat, green vegetables and dried fruit. If your iron count is low, your doctor will give you an iron supplement to boost your intake.

ZINC

This mineral helps to promote healthy growth and brain and nerve formation. It may also prevent morning sickness. A deficiency of the mineral during pregnancy can lead to restricted foetal growth. Zinc is found in all meat and fish and is present in plant seeds, such as sesame and sunflower seeds, wheat and oat germ and sprouts such as alfalfa. To be certain of a sufficient zinc intake, you and your partner should start taking a zinc supplement a few months before you intend to conceive. A good daily intake is from 15 to 20mg. You'll double your absorption of the mineral if you take it with vitamin B6 – but try to avoid drinking coffee after taking it as this can halve the amount of zinc you'll actually absorb.

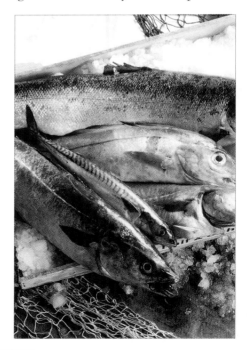

VITAMIN B12

If you're a vegetarian and worried about getting enough of the right nutrients, it's well worth taking a vitamin B12 supplement. This vitamin helps to form haemoglobin and the baby's central nervous system, and is mainly found in meat, fish and poultry, although wholegrain cereals and dairy products also contain it.

FISH OIL

A regular intake of fish oil may benefit you and your baby during the pregnancy. The best source of this oil is in dark fish such as herring and mackerel, but if you don't like fish, you can take fish oil supplements such as cod liver oil. Fish oil contains substances which are not found in any other oil – EPA (eicosapentaenoic acid) and DHA (docosahexaenoic acid). These essential fatty acids have been shown to reduce the tendency of blood to clot, thus reducing the risk of thrombosis. They also reduce blood pressure and improve kidney function. DHA is needed for brain development and is particularly important for premature babies as the major development in a baby's brain occurs during the last three months of pregnancy.

It is also advisable to increase your intake of other important vitamins and minerals, such as vitamins B1 (thiamine), B2 (riboflavin), B3 (niacin), B5 (pantothenic acid), B6 (pyridoxine), biotin and vitamin D. These B vitamins are needed to enable us to get the energy we need from food and they can be bought together in a vitamin B-complex supplement. Biotin promotes healthy hair and nail growth, while vitamin D works with calcium to build healthy blood and strong bones.

OTHER PRECAUTIONS

CUT BACK ON CAFFEINE

Caffeine is an addictive stimulant which can over-activate the nervous system. Drinking coffee or tea can cause the heartbeat to speed up and could have a similar effect on your baby, as caffeine can cross the placenta. Drinking coffee and tea with or after meals can also prevent you from absorbing vital vitamins and minerals. For example, if you drink tea during a meal, you're reducing your absorption of iron, and if you drink coffee after a meal you can halve the amount of zinc you've absorbed from your food. There are many alternatives to caffeine, such as the huge range of delicious herbal teas currently available. Dandelion and chicory coffees are also useful alternatives.

SMOKING

If either you or your partner smoke it could hinder your chances of conceiving. Smoking reduces the levels of vitamin C in the body and a study by Professor Bruce Ames of the University of California has found a clear link between low levels of this vitamin and genetically damaged sperm. Smoking damages DNA by oxidation and so causes genetic damage that could be inherited.

Female smokers are damaging their chances of having a child further, as maternal smoking can cause problems such as slow development of the foetus in the uterus leading to spontaneous abortion, premature birth or low infant birthweight. A report from the Royal College of Physicians, *Health or Smoking*, concluded that, 'Women who smoke are more likely to be infertile or take longer to conceive than women who do not smoke.' The Royal College of Physicians also found that over 4,000 miscarriages of healthy foetuses occur because of maternal smoking during pregnancy. In its report, *Smoking and the Young*, the Royal College concluded that maternal smoking during pregnancy and infancy is 'the most important avoidable risk factor for infant death'.

THINK BEFORE YOU DRINK

Medical opinion varies on how safe it is for pregnant women to drink. A heavy intake of alcohol (eight glasses of wine a day or the equivalent) has been shown to affect fertility and can damage the unborn child. Ten percent of babies born to heavy drinkers may suffer from foetal alcohol syndrome (FAS). These children have a receding forehead and chin and suffer from various behavioural and developmental problems as they grow older. While some doctors advise that you cut out alcohol completely while you are pregnant, others say that 'moderate' drinking is safe for the unborn baby. Moderate drinking is usually described as one or two alcoholic units once or twice a week. Drinking wine is thought to be less harmful than beer, because the latter contains thiocyanate, also found in tobacco.

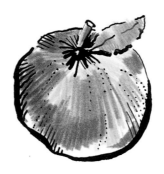

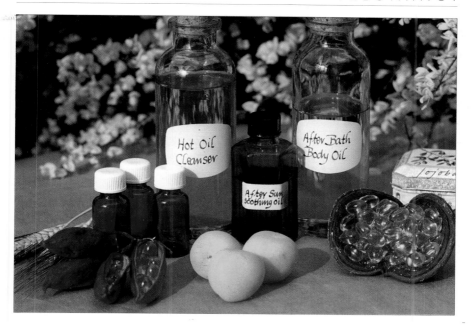

NATURAL PREGNANCY
REMEDY FINDER

BACK PAIN

Low backache is very common in pregnancy. You are using different muscles in your lower back from those you would normally use and this often leads to muscle strain.

Ask your partner to massage your back with an oil mixture containing 10 drops of one or more of any of the following essential oils: sandalwood, citrus, geranium and patchouli – ten drops per 50ml base oil such as grapeseed or almond.

For muscular tension, try drinking relaxing teas such as chamomile and lemon balm. Also try massaging your lower back with a few drops of lavender essential oil, mixed in 50ml of a base oil, such as almond or grapeseed. (Essential oils are too concentrated to be used neat on the skin. For massage they should be mixed with a carrier oil.)

CONSTIPATION

Very common in pregnancy as food moves at a slower rate through the intestines, due to the relaxing effect of your pregnancy hormones which decrease the muscle tone of the bowels. Your growing uterus also takes up more space which was previously occupied by your intestines, causing your digestive system to slow down even more. Constipation can also sometimes be caused by taking an iron supplement.

Make sure you're eating plenty of fibre – from fruit, vegetables and wholegrains (apart from wheat). Try to cut out bread and wheat products for a while as they can have a blocking effect. Drink lots of fluids, avoid using laxatives and try taking vitamin C supplements (3–5g per day). Drinking hot water or tea with lemon as soon as you wake up, and waiting half an hour before you eat anything else, may also stimulate your bowels. A few spoonfuls of linseeds taken with a large glass or two of water or fruit juice, or sprinkled onto cereal or yoghurt, also help to regulate the bowels. Some herbs can be made into teas to stimulate the bowels without irritation such as chamomile and dandelion root.

EXHAUSTION / FATIGUE

You will probably feel very tired in early pregnancy, more energetic in the middle months and need plenty of rest in the last three months. But continuous tiredness is unusual and may be connected to anaemia or anxiety.

Soak in a warm bath with one drop of mandarin, one drop of reviving ylang-ylang and two drops of rosewood essential oil.

Get as much rest as you feel you need and eat a well-balanced diet. Try to keep up some form of gentle exercise such as yoga or swimming. Supplement your diet with a multivitamin and mineral tonic and a B-vitamin complex. In later pregnancy, rosemary tea is very good. For anxiety drink chamomile tea, and for exhaustion, try cinnamon tea.

MORNING SICKNESS / NAUSEA

Many women experience this in the first three or four months of pregnancy, but some suffer for the entire nine months. Various factors are thought to cause nausea including low blood sugar, low blood pressure and hormonal changes.

Place a drop of peppermint oil on a handkerchief and inhale. Get out of bed slowly and have a drink with a dry biscuit or piece of toast on waking. Instead of tea or coffee, drink a glass of hot lemon and honey or a cup of herbal tea – try lemon balm, chamomile, raspberry leaf, peppermint or fennel tea. Eat small amounts of food about six times a day. If you've lost your appetite, take a vitamin B6 supplement. Ginger is an excellent remedy for morning sickness. Take up to 1g of the powdered herb in a capsule or two to five drops of the tincture in water or under the

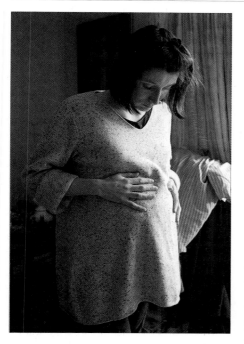

tongue. Drinking ginger beer or eating ginger biscuits is also said to help!

VARICOSE VEINS

Small veins in your legs may swell up, become painful and show during pregnancy. This is because the volume of blood increases when you're pregnant, which stretches the walls and the valves in the veins. This can cause blood to gather in the lower limbs – resulting in varicose veins.

Try to avoid standing for long periods and do regular exercise to maintain your muscle tone. Splash your legs with cold water – this will help alleviate soreness of inflamed veins. Make sure you sit with your feet up for a short time each day. Support tights are also very useful, but need to be put on *before* you stand up – so keep a pair beside the bed and wriggle into them in the morning!

STRETCH MARKS

These long red streaks are a problem everyone associates with pregnancy – fortunately, after the birth they fade to a pale silvery colour. Stretch marks may appear over your tummy, breasts and buttocks as dark or reddish streaks towards the end of pregnancy, showing that the skin has been stretched from underneath. They are more common in fair-skinned and overweight women, although who gets stretch marks is largely a question of luck and genetics. But, by using oils or creams to rub into your skin, you may avoid getting them. There are some commercial stretch-mark creams available, but you can actually use any oil or cream which is easily absorbed into your skin. Try a daily massage using almond or vitamin E oil or one of the rich vitamin E creams available. A healthy diet rich in vitamins C and E and zinc will help to build strong skin from within.

EXERCISE

Exercise helps our circulation and digestion and even helps to stimulate the mind. Regular exercise will also help you to prepare yourself for the birth – by strengthening and toning your muscles. Staying fit will help you to stop putting on too much weight and may give you more energy – believe it or not – exercise can make you feel less tired! You may also avoid getting some of the typical pregnancy problems such as varicose veins and cramp. In addition, regular physical activity will make it easier for you to relax and sleep at night.

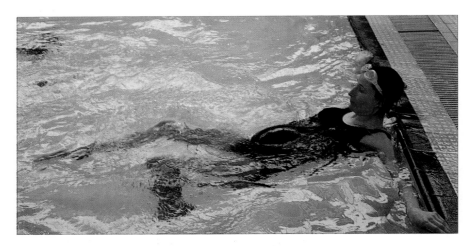

Walking and swimming are the two best forms of aerobic exercise for pregnancy. Try walking briskly three times each week for 15 to 30 minutes and swim gentle lengths at your local pool – any stroke is fine. If you've enjoyed cycling or tennis before your pregnancy – keep it up – but it's not a particularly good time to start these from scratch. Yoga is an excellent activity to take up at this time, as it can teach you useful stretching and breathing exercises, which may prove invaluable during the birth. It will also help you relieve stress and allow your body to become more supple.

HOW TO EXERCISE SAFELY DURING PREGNANCY

☐ Never overdo things. If you begin to feel tired, dizzy or strained – stop immediately.

☐ Warm up properly before you begin and give yourself a chance to cool down and wind down afterwards.

☐ Make sure you don't overheat
– it's not good for you or the
baby.

☐ Don't get dehydrated – drink
as much water as you need,
before and after.

☐ Seek your doctor's advice
before starting any exercise
programme.

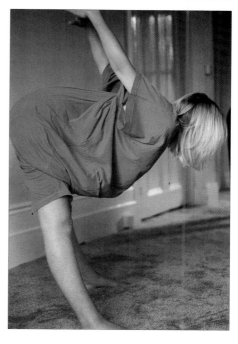

PELVIC FLOOR EXERCISES A vital
exercise – not just for birth – but
for life! The pelvic floor is a very
important group of muscles, yet
many women know very little
about them. These muscles lie at
the bottom of the pelvis,
supporting the womb, bladder
and bowels – rather like a
hammock. The pelvic floor is
shaped rather like a figure of
eight, with a large loop which controls the urethra and vagina and a
smaller ring at the back, controlling the anal sphincter. These two rings
overlap in the centre – called the perineum.

If your pelvic floor weakens, you can suffer from a minor leak of urine
each time you cough, laugh, sneeze or run for the bus. During birth these
muscles are particularly important, as the pelvic floor has to relax and
stretch to allow the baby to pass through the vaginal opening. After the
birth the pelvic floor may weaken, so it's well worth exercising these
muscles during pregnancy. To find out where your pelvic floor actually is,
try stopping yourself next time you are urinating. Just stop mid-stream
and hold briefly – then empty your bladder. It's the muscles you use to
stop the flow that you should be using in pelvic floor exercises.

When you've established where the muscle is, try doing this simple
exercise every day. Choose a position you feel comfortable in – it may be
lying on your back with your knees up, or just sitting on a chair. Now
slowly pull yourself in and tighten up from around the back passage
through to the middle and then the front. Try to hold for four to five
counts and then let go. Aim to do five to ten at first and then gradually
build up until you're doing 50 or more each day. You can do this exercise
anywhere, any time!

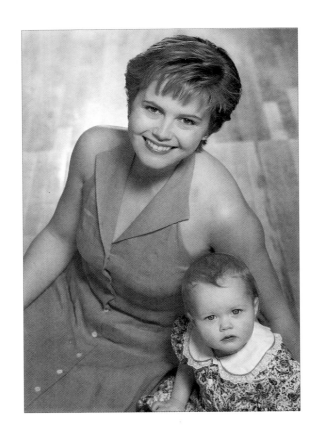

6

Postnatal

Having a baby changes your life. Not only in the practical aspect of becoming somebody's parent, but also on many mental, emotional and physical levels. It may take a while to appreciate that you have actually become a parent. You are now responsible for a small baby – something which you may never have experienced before. You are to clothe, feed and care for a tiny human being who is totally dependent on you. You now have a full-time commitment to your new child.

YOUR HEALTH

If you had a demanding and exhausting birth, you may feel that it is you who needs plenty of care and attention – not just your baby. Try to relax. Making sure you have as much help as you can during the first couple of weeks at home to look after your baby and do some housework can really make a difference in the difficult transition to motherhood. Take up every offer from grandparents, friends and neighbours! To help relax your exhausted mind and body, have a couple of warm baths each day. Try adding a couple of drops of your favourite essential oil to the bath water. Lavender and/or sandalwood essential oils are particularly soothing and relaxing.

In the first few days after the birth you may be in pain because of stitches which can make it difficult for you to go to the loo. However, it is important to pass water regularly. If you feel a stinging or burning sensation in your vaginal area as you pass water, keep a bottle or jug filled with cold water next to the toilet to pour between your legs each time you

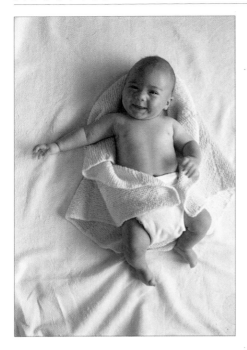

empty your bladder. Instead of drying yourself with a paper towel you may prefer to use a hairdryer for the first day or so (remember not to use your hairdryer in the bathroom). Also, try the tips already mentioned on page 66 to help prevent constipation. Taking the homeopathic remedy of Arnica 30C tablets every four hours for the first few days can significantly reduce any bruising and speed the healing process.

After the birth, your uterus continues to contract until it reaches its former size. As a result, you may feel mild period-type pains or have stronger, more uncomfortable twinges. With your first baby, you will probably feel very little, but the after-pains can get worse with each subsequent birth as your uterus has to work harder to contract back to its previous size. Although uncomfortable, this means that your body will get back into shape more quickly.

After the birth, you may feel incredibly light and sylph-like – having lost the weight of the baby, the placenta and water. But you may be a little surprised that you don't immediately return to your pre-pregnant shape. Your tummy will look a little saggy and you may still be quite a lot larger than you were before you became pregnant. This is partly because your muscles have stretched. However, if you eat a balanced diet and start doing some gentle abdominal exercises, your pre-pregnancy figure will return.

POSTNATAL EXERCISES

If you've had a Caesarean you shouldn't start doing any of these exercises (apart from the pelvic floor exercise) for at least a few weeks after the birth. Your doctor or midwife will tell you when you're ready to start. It is a good idea for all postnatal women to do some pelvic floor exercises after the birth (see page 69). A few weeks after the birth you can start to do more strenuous exercise such as yoga and swimming. These forms of exercise are both excellent for helping you return to your former shape.

A few days after the birth you can begin to exercise your stomach muscles:

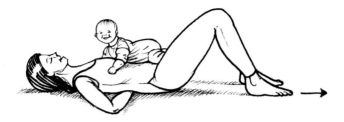

Lying in the same position, breathe out, and push the floor or the bed with your feet. Let your pelvis roll in, so your lower back flattens. Gently push the floor or bed with your feet, so your pelvis rolls and lets your lower back arch. If you unfold your arms and let them lie on the floor while you do this, you can do this exercise with your baby lying on your stomach!

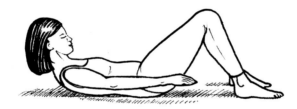

Lie on the floor with legs bent and arms at your sides. Tighten your abdominal muscles. Then, bringing your chin to your chest, curl up as far as you can, gradually stretching your hands to your feet. Slowly lower yourself back to the floor.

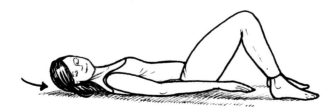

Lie on the floor with your legs bent, arms by your sides. Tighten your abdominal muscles and slowly raise your head and shoulders. As you do this, slide your right hand to touch your right foot and bend sideways. Then straighten up and repeat on your left-hand side.

BABY BLUES

You may feel on a complete high immediately after giving birth, and find it difficult to sleep for the first couple of nights. However, this elation may give way to feeling very weepy between the third and fifth day after you've had the baby. You may worry about small problems or frequently burst into tears. This is quite normal – as your body and emotions have been through a huge upheaval and you're bound to want to cry a little.

Baby blues can be caused by fatigue, hormonal changes, pain from stitches or sore breasts or simply a feeling of anticlimax after the build-up to the birth. Often, all that is needed is some rest or a good cry. Talk about your feelings to your partner, friends or midwife. The baby blues should only last for a day or two – so if it lasts for longer or becomes more of a depression, seek help as soon as possible.

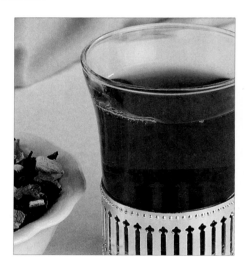

There are a number of lifestyle changes that can help relieve postnatal depression. Firstly, make sure your diet has plenty of healthy raw fruits and vegetables and eat protein frequently. Eating little and often will help you to maintain blood-sugar levels making you less likely to feel angry or depressed. Drink plenty of fluids and cut out caffeine as it may be making you feel irritable and anxious – try herbal teas such as camomile, fennel and peppermint instead. It is a good idea to take some form of exercise every day, even if you just walk to the shops with baby and pushchair. Just getting out of your home and seeing some other people can help you feel better.

An alternative therapy, such as aromatherapy, can also help alleviate depression. Choose a couple of essential oils you really like and put a few drops in a hot bath, then soak for a long time. Oils which aromatherapists say can help relieve depression include bergamot, clary sage, geranium, jasmine, neroli, rose, sandalwood, tangerine and ylang-ylang. Or make up a massage oil using some of these oils and ask your partner or a friend to give you a really soothing massage. To make your own inhalation, mix together 20 drops of clary sage and 10 drops of rose and store the mixture in a dark glass bottle. Each morning and evening, sprinkle a few drops on a tissue and inhale. You can try the same mix in a room vaporiser, for an uplifting effect.

BREASTFEEDING

After your baby is born, your breasts will appear very much larger. For the first few days after the birth, they secrete a special food called colostrum. This yellowish liquid contains the antibodies your baby needs to help protect him or her from illness and disease. It is richer in protein than your later milk and helps the baby to sleep for long periods in between feeds. This may be nature's way of giving you a rest after a tiring birth! Even if you do not intend to breastfeed, it is well worth giving your baby this very special elixir as a nutritious start to life.

If your baby sucks on the colostrum, your milk will come in between the second to the sixth day after you've given birth. However, If you decide not to breastfeed, you will be prescribed medication to suppress the normal milk production and your breasts will return to their normal size about a week later. If you do decide to breastfeed, your breasts will probably feel very full when the milk arrives and you may even have the sensation that you're about to burst. This fullness is called engorgement and usually disappears in a couple of days. If your breasts are engorged, feed your baby frequently as it's important to empty the breast and relieve this feeling. A warm bath or shower followed by a feed may help to reduce engorgement. Also, try placing very hot flannels around the breasts and use gentle massage strokes towards the nipples to help clear blocked milk ducts. The amount of milk you produce will gradually regulate itself according to the quantity needed by your baby and you will lose the uncomfortably full feeling. Your breasts may leak for the first few days after your milk has come in, so try wearing breast pads inside your bra to pick up the runaway droplets.

THE BENEFITS OF BREASTFEEDING

Human milk contains essential fatty acids which can help your baby's physical and mental development. Your milk is also good for your baby's brain and blood vessel growth, while protecting him or her from coughs, colds, chest and stomach infections. Some studies have even shown that breastfed babies are marginally more intelligent and have a higher IQ rating than bottle-fed babies. This is possibly due to the presence in breast milk of these essential fatty acids needed for brain development. There is some evidence to show that breastfed babies are less likely to get allergies or develop certain diseases in later life. Breastfed babies are also unlikely to become constipated and their stools are soft and not as smelly as those of bottle-fed babies.

Breastfeeding is also good for you. Statistics show that breastfeeding reduces a woman's risk of developing breast cancer later on in life. Considering that one in nine women develop breast cancer, this is a significant factor in the decision whether to breastfeed or not. Breastfeeding will also help to establish a special bond between you and your baby. It even helps you to regain your former figure more quickly by stimulating your uterus to contract after the birth.

BEGINNING BREASTFEEDING

You can tell if your baby is correctly positioned for breastfeeding if there is more of your areola (the darker coloured area surrounding your nipple) showing above the baby's top lip than below the bottom. Your baby's gums should be working on the areola, not dragging on your nipple, which should be at the back of the mouth. You should neither lean back nor too far forward when breastfeeding as this makes it more difficult for your baby to latch onto your breast. If feeding hurts or your baby doesn't seem to be getting enough milk, you may be badly positioned, so stop the feed by putting your little finger in the corner of his or her mouth. Then alter your feeding position and start again.

ESSENTIAL EXTRAS

Bear in mind that your requirements for most vitamins and minerals dramatically increase during breastfeeding, so a well-balanced multi-vitamin and mineral formula would be worth taking. Other nutrients can help to boost your energy supplies and relieve postnatal depression.

B-complex vitamins: Research has shown that a lack of B vitamins and calcium can lead to fatigue and irritability, so it is worth taking these as supplements to try and prevent the problem.

Iodine: If you find yourself lacking in energy, taking iodine supplements may help as this essential trace mineral controls the speed at which we burn oxygen to provide energy. Eating little and often can also help to boost your energy levels.

Iron: As you lose blood in the first couple of weeks after the birth, it may be advisable to take an iron supplement to replace that which is lost as a result. To help your body absorb iron, try eating more vitamin C-rich foods, such as citrus fruits, broccoli, potatoes and cabbage.

Zinc: If you're breastfeeding it is worth taking a zinc supplement as you need plenty of the mineral to aid your baby's development. One study found that the zinc content of food eaten by pregnant and breastfeeding

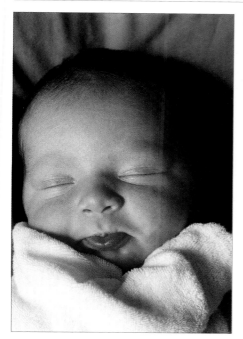

women only provided 42 percent of the recommended daily allowance. A good daily intake is from 15 to 20mg (make sure you take the elemental as opposed to the compound zinc). Try to avoid drinking coffee after taking zinc as this can halve the amount you actually absorb.

Folic acid: You may be short of folic acid – vital for normal cell function and the production of red blood cells. You can either buy a supplement or find it in dry beans and fresh green vegetables such as spinach and lettuce. You will absorb folic acid more easily if you eat plenty of vitamin C and vitamin B-rich foods.

Calcium, magnesium and phosphorus: It is especially important that you increase your intake of these three minerals if you are breastfeeding, as they are essential for building strong, healthy teeth and bones.

Antioxidants: You also need an increased intake of the antioxidant nutrients to help to build your baby's immune system. These include vitamin C, beta-carotene, vitamin E, selenium and copper.

EXPRESS YOURSELF

A few weeks after the birth, you may want to leave your baby with a friend or relative so you can have a much needed break. If you're breastfeeding, the best way to provide for your baby in this time is to express some milk from your breasts. Learning to express can be like learning to breastfeed all over again. One option is to buy a hand or battery operated breast pump, which can be quicker than expressing milk by hand. Electric pumps can also be hired from your local branch of the National Childbirth Trust or La Lèche League (see Useful Addresses). The breast pump works in the same way as your baby's mouth by stimulating your milk ducts to express milk.

Some women find expressing by hand is far easier (and cheaper) than using a pump. There are several ways of doing this. Firstly, sterilise a bowl to catch the milk as it comes out. You can try warming your breasts by applying hot flannels and then massaging your breast for a few minutes. Work your way around the breast, starting from the top and moving round to the bottom. Do this about ten times to encourage your milk to flow. Then stroke your breasts with a downwards motion towards the areola a couple of times. Using your thumb and forefingers, squeeze your nipple, while pressing backwards at the same time. The milk should now begin to spurt out into the bowl. Continue to squeeze your breast until it only expresses a few drops, squeezing different parts of the breast so you empty the milk ducts properly. Then move to the other breast and follow the same procedure.

When you have enough milk for a feed, store it in a sterilised, capped bottle in the fridge. But don't keep it for more than twenty-four hours, or it will go off. To keep milk for a few weeks, you can freeze it in special freezer bags, available from chemists, the National Childbirth Trust (NCT) and La Lèche League. When you need the milk, put it in the fridge until completely defrosted, but don't try to warm it up until it has thawed.

BOTTLE FEEDING

If you can't or simply don't want to breastfeed, bottle feeding is the answer. Make sure you have at least six bottles and teats, a supply of formula milk and sterilising equipment. Follow the instructions on the formula packet exactly – any extra could harm your baby. You can store ready-prepared bottles in the fridge for up to twenty-four hours. Sterilise each bottle and teat before use with chemical sterilising tablets or liquid in cold water, or by using a steam steriliser.

When bottle feeding, you should hold your baby close and let him or her have as much milk as s/he wants. After each feed throw away any leftover milk. Make sure that you keep the bottle tilted so the teat is full of milk or your baby will take in air. If s/he seems unhappy with the bottle, try a different kind of teat. They are available in lots of different shapes and sizes – even nipple-shaped! Never leave your baby alone with a bottle in his or her mouth, or add solids to the milk, as this can cause choking.

STARTING ON SOLIDS

Most babies are given their first mouthfuls of solid food between the ages of four and six months. Before a baby is three months old, his or her digestive system isn't capable of absorbing foods more complex than baby-milk. It is now thought that the later you leave the introduction of solids the better. Your baby will probably start to show signs indicating when s/he is ready for solids, such as demanding more feeds.

When you start to give your baby its first few mouthfuls of solids, breast or formula milk should continue to be the main source of nutrition and milk feeds should not be reduced. The new food should be introduced in the middle or at the end of a milk feed, as s/he will be more receptive to the idea once the initial hunger pangs have been satisfied. For the first two weeks, just give the solids to your baby once a day, and gradually build up until you are giving solids at three feeds a day.

Start with a small plastic teaspoon of thin porridge made from oat flakes, rice flakes or cornmeal, mixed with a little breast or formula milk. Commercial baby rice is another great starter food and is very convenient. Most brands are nutritionally sound, but check first that the baby rice you use is completely salt and sugar free. You can offer your baby some new flavours after a couple of weeks, but leave a few days in between each new flavour as taste is a new experience for a baby. This will also give you the chance to look out for any allergic reaction to food in the form of diarrhoea or skin rashes. Try offering a little vegetable or fruit purée – without any salt or sugar. You could try potato, carrot, parsnip, plantain, broccoli, spinach, pear, apple or banana. If your baby refuses a food – don't force it – just try again a couple of weeks later, when s/he may be more enthusiastic.

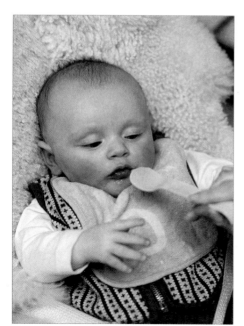

WHAT FOODS TO AVOID

Don't give your baby any salt, sugar or fatty foods. And avoid all of the following: milk apart from breast or formula milk, all other dairy products including cheese, eggs, wheat-based foods such as wheat cereals and pasta, citrus fruits and summer fruits such as strawberries and raspberries. These can produce an allergic reaction, so are better left until the baby is a few months older. Also avoid tomatoes, spices, chillies and nuts. For more comprehensive information on weaning, read my *Quick Guide to Baby and Toddler Foods* (Boxtree).

COMMON BABY AILMENTS

COLIC

This is a problem faced by many parents in the first few months and usually happens after feeding. A colicky baby will cry and may draw his or her legs up or stretch them right out as if in pain. There is still disagreement about what colic really is, but it is thought to be sharp abdominal pains or cramps caused by wind. Colic is sometimes used as a term for a baby who simply cries a lot for no particular reason. Some babies do just cry a great deal and can be inconsolable – but this problem does resolve itself when the baby reaches three or four months – so don't feel as if it is your fault. Both breastfed and bottlefed babies can suffer from colic.

To prevent colic always wind your baby after a feed, by sitting him or her up on your knee and gently patting the back, or by leaning him or her over your shoulder. Try giving your baby a bottle of cooled, boiled water if you think he or she is thirsty rather than hungry. Comfort your baby – perhaps by gentle rocking or even putting him or her in a sling and walking around the house.

NAPPY RASH

If the area around your baby's genitals become spotty, red and sore, then he or she probably has nappy rash. This is usually caused by leaving your baby's nappy on for too long, so change it regularly, cleaning and drying his or her bottom thoroughly. Whenever you can, let your baby lie around without a nappy to expose him or her to the air. If you're using terry nappies, don't use a biological powder or fabric conditioner to clean them as these can cause an allergic reaction. Use a good barrier cream and nappy rash cream.

THRUSH

This is an infection caused by a yeast which lives in the mouth and intestines and is common in young babies. It is usually kept under control by bacteria but it can get out of hand, producing an irritating rash. Your baby has oral thrush if you can see white patches on the tongue or inside his or her cheeks. These may look like bits of milk, but don't come off if wiped with a cloth. To avoid oral thrush, wash your nipples carefully after each breastfeed, as they can become infected. Don't use soap on them – just water. Don't wear breast pads. If you are bottle feeding, buy a special soft teat and clean it carefully and sterilise after each feed.

Genital thrush is often confused with nappy rash. The main difference is that while thrush usually starts around the anus and spreads outwards, sometimes up to the tummy button, nappy rash will begin in the baby's creases. To alleviate genital thrush don't use bubble bath in your baby's baths and stop using plastic pants over your baby's nappies until the rash has cleared. Let as much fresh air as possible get to your baby's bottom. Consult your doctor if the problem persists.

TEETHING

Your baby may cut his or her first tooth, usually in the front at the bottom – at any time during the first year – although the average age is five to six months. Some babies may suffer pain from sore, swollen gums, as well as having colds, coughs, earache, diarrhoea and sleeplessness as a result. You may be able to see where your baby's gum is sore and red where the tooth is about to come through, or that one cheek is flushed. Rubbing your baby's gums with a finger will often help ease the pain. Giving your baby something hard to chew, such as a teething ring, can also help. Try to avoid giving your baby too many doses of medicines or teething gels and avoid rusks because they all contain sugar. Even at this stage, constant chewing and sucking on sugary things can cause tooth decay. My babies gnawed happily on pieces of bread baked hard in a cool oven for several hours, but sometimes it is hard to tell whether chewing is due to teething.

COPING WITH CRYING

Most new-born babies cry a lot – often to the distraction of their parents who simply cannot find a way to soothe them. This is often simply due to tiredness, and putting your fractious baby in his or her cot can often solve the problem. You can also try carrying your baby around in a sling as the rocking motion will help to soothe him or her and may encourage sleep! Another way to calm your baby down is to wrap him or her tightly in a shawl, so the arms and legs are restricted. This often calms a baby down and is very effective for babies up to two months old. It is also important to cuddle your baby as s/he needs plenty of affection and loving.

If your baby's crying gets too much for you, leave him or her with a friend or relative for an hour just to give yourself a break. There are organisations which offer support for parents of crying babies. One such group, Cry-sis, has branches in different areas and will put you in touch with other mothers who have had the same problem (see Useful Addresses).

Note: Crying can be a sign of illness. If your baby's cry sounds different from normal, or there is something unusual about the way your baby is behaving, then contact your doctor immediately.

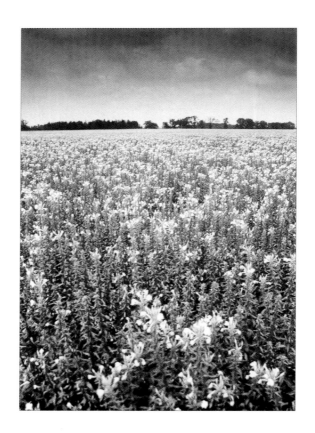

7

Menopause

T he menopause occurs at what we generally call 'middle age' which can be a time of great upheaval in many people's lives. For a mother, this is often the age at which her children have grownup and left home. For those who have gone in for motherhood later in life, the menopause may come at a time when their children are in mid-puberty and enduring the throes of their first hormonal upheaval. For childless women, the menopause is the time to come to terms with the fact that natural motherhood is no longer possible. We may all have to come to terms with disappointments at this stage in our lives, but it is important not to allow them to interfere with the many potential joys yet to come.

The changes of the menopause do not occur suddenly, but develop over a number of years. These changes are brought about by our hormones – chemicals made by various glands in the body. During the menopause the regular monthly cycle of menstruation brought about by the hormones oestrogen and progesterone finishes. 'Menopause' actually means a woman's last period, and we don't know exactly when this has occurred until a year or two has passed to prove that it was indeed the last. This is because our periods become infrequent during the years running up to the menopause. This slowing-down process can take up to five years. It is known technically as 'the climacteric' and has three stages:

Stage one: The 'pre-menopause' is the time when the periods first begin to be less regular in their timing and vary in their degree of heaviness.
Stage two: The 'peri-menopause' includes the years when other physical

and sometimes psychological alterations are noticed. During the peri-menopause, the true menopause occurs, and the final period is experienced.

Stage three: The 'post-menopause' covers the years after the menopause, beginning with the menopause itself and lasting the rest of our days.

The menopause usually begins between the ages of forty-five and fifty, although it is not unusual for it to start at forty. When the first signs appear, it is a good idea to make a note of the start date of each period and its duration. This will show how regular or irregular, light or heavy each is. If a woman is over fifty and has had no period for a whole year, the menopause is considered to be complete. However, in women under fifty, it is wise to allow two years and continue using contraception before making any assumptions!

SYMPTOMS OF THE MENOPAUSE

There is much more to the menopause than merely the end of menstruation. If this was the only symptom, I doubt that it would cause much concern! Unfortunately, around 80 percent of women experience additional symptoms, the majority of which can be easily relieved.

HOT FLUSHES AND NIGHT SWEATS

Hot flushes and the associated night sweats are a symptom of the peri-menopausal phase. It seems that the hormones involved in bringing on the menopause also have an effect on the way in which the body controls temperature. The body's thermostat becomes set too low, telling us that we are too cold. So the body reacts by expanding the blood vessels, allowing more blood to flow to the skin, causing it to redden and heat up. We then perspire to cool down these overheated areas, which gives rise to anything from a slight clamminess to rivulets of sweat. Hot flushes are often accompanied by a sudden increase in heart rate and blood pressure which explains why they can cause anxiety and feelings of exhaustion.

Fortunately, hot flushes can be reduced by taking HRT or by balancing hormones naturally with a daily dose of evening primrose oil. Taking time over your meals so that they can be fully digested can also help. Spicy foods, hot drinks, alcohol, sugar, caffeine, which is found in tea and chocolate as well as coffee, can all bring on hot flushes. Smoking has a bad effect on the circulation and thus intensifies both hot flushes and night sweats, so there is yet another good reason for giving it up. Regular exercise helps to boost circulation and so helps to prevent hot flushes. Your weight can also influence whether or not you will suffer from these dreaded sweats. Aim to be neither too fat nor too thin. Thin women are more likely to have hot flushes than those who are slightly overweight, because fatty tissue is a source of oestrogen that thin women do not have. It is thought that hot flushes are caused by a lack of oestrogen and it is true that in Japan where the diet contains many oestrogen-rich foods, women do not suffer from hot flushes – in fact, they do not even have a name for them.

Wear cotton clothing rather than nylon or polyester to allow your skin to breathe more easily. Cotton bed sheets may also help to reduce night sweats. A fan kept beside the bed is useful in keeping you cool at night as is a bowl of tepid, not cold, water and a flannel for sponging down the face, neck and chest. If sleep is so disturbed by night sweats that it is impossible to get a good night's rest, or hot flushes are seriously interfering with daily life, causing depression and exhaustion, seek professional help. You may be prescribed Hormone Replacement Therapy (HRT – see page 89). It is also helpful to keep a diary of both hot flushes and night sweats to see if a pattern develops. It may then be possible to avoid certain situations or foods that trigger them.

OSTEOPOROSIS

Bone mass is constantly being broken down and remade and when we are still in the growth stage of life, the rebuilding of healthy bones is going on faster than the breaking down part of the process. As we get older the situation reverses, resulting in the weakening of our bones – allowing fractures to occur more easily. This thinning of the bone is referred to as osteoporosis.

Fortunately, it is possible to halt the thinning of our bones, although the condition can pass unnoticed for several years. Osteoporosis can start when we are only in our mid-thirties and its effects may be invisible for a decade or so. The first symptoms are often back pain. If you cannot stand for as long as you would like without developing back-ache, especially in the lower back, it can be a sign that the bones are thinning. Only later would the breaks and eventual deformity of the 'dowager's hump' occur, caused by the crumbling of the vertebrae. A slight reduction in height is another important symptom.

Diet and exercise play an important role in preventing osteoporosis. Calcium, in particular, is recognised as holding the key to healthy, strong bones in later life. We can excrete up to 900mg of calcium each day and this needs to be replaced. Menopausal women need an increased supply of this vital mineral as calcium absorption decreases with age. Experts advise that menopausal women and the elderly have a daily intake of between 1,000mg and 1,500mg of calcium. Good sources of calcium include hard cheese such as cheddar, milk, low-fat plain yoghurt, spinach, watercress, canned fish, canned beans or peas, tofu and green leafy vegetables. If you do not eat a lot of these foods it is worth supplementing your diet.

Alcohol, caffeine and nicotine all interfere with calcium absorption and so should be avoided. Calcium works together with magnesium and vitamin D to maintain healthy bones. Magnesium is required to activate vitamin D which in turn aids calcium absorption. We should, therefore, also increase our intake of these nutrients. Cod liver oil is the best source of vitamin D, but it can also be found in eggs and milk. Our bodies also produce their own supply of vitamin D through exposure to sunlight. Magnesium is mainly found in soya beans, nuts, wholewheat flour, wholemeal bread and pasta, seafood and green vegetables.

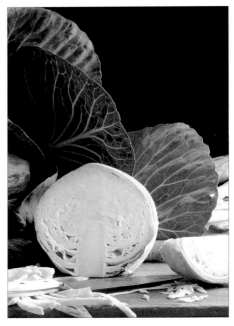

SKIN PROBLEMS

We tend to think of our skin as our outermost layer, but the most important part of it lies a few millimetres beneath the surface – the connective tissue. Our skin grows and replaces itself every few weeks from this base layer and it is to this we need to pay the most attention. Helping the skin in the continual process of renewal are the blood vessels, fat cells, hair follicles and nerve endings. Also necessary to all this activity are the hormones and oxygen which are transported throughout the body via blood circulation. Oestrogen is needed to keep our skin firm and youthful and during the menopause the level of oestrogen in the skin drops dramatically. From our mid-thirties onwards the whole renewal process slows down; the fat cells are reduced and the collagen and elastin present in the connective tissue become weaker. The weakening of this support system causes the skin to loosen and wrinkle. The replacement of skin cells also slows down, so that the dead surface cells remain on the body for longer, becoming drier through over-exposure to the elements.

But, depressing as this sounds, there is still much which can be done to improve the condition of our skin with a healthy diet full of fresh fruit and vegetable and wholegrains to supply our bodies with the skin-saving antioxidants. If you smoke, give it up *now* as it is the number one enemy of healthy skin. It increases wrinkling and reduces our circulation by narrowing the blood vessels, starving the skin of nutrients and suffocating it with a lack of oxygen. Overexposure to sunlight also damages our skin and increases wrinkling so wear high factor sunscreens when exposed to its harsh rays.

One of the many benefits of HRT is that it can significantly improve the condition of our skin. According to research carried out by a leading consultant gynaecologist in London, Dr John Studd, taking HRT results in a 30 percent increase in skin thickness and a 34 percent increase in the amount of collagen in the skin making it significantly firmer. A daily dose of evening primrose oil may help improve menopausal skin as it helps to balance our hormone levels naturally. The essential fatty acids in evening primrose oil also help to maintain the water barrier that helps to keep our skin moist and supple.

VAGINAL DRYNESS

The reduction of secretions affecting the visible areas of our skin is also at work unseen. A very vulnerable spot is the vagina and the area of skin immediately around it. The resulting dryness can make sexual intercourse uncomfortable and even painful and this often results in a reluctance to have sex. Unfortunately the effect of this is to cut off the supply of the natural lubrication released during lovemaking. Not unnaturally, this can cause tension and depression which in turn inhibits the production of natural lubricants and the whole thing becomes a vicious circle.

Vaginal dryness can be helped by the liberal use of lubricants. Avoid creams containing petroleum jelly, especially if you are using condoms or a diaphragm for contraception as these cause the latex to disintegrate. Also avoid using perfumed soaps, scented bath oils, talcum powders, shower gels and lotions.

BREAST PROBLEMS

Just as a woman's breasts develop during the hormonal changes of puberty, they change again during the menopause. Oestrogen depletion weakens the supporting tissues of the whole body and so the breasts tend to sag under their own weight.

Another breast problem some women experience during the menopause is breast pain in the form of mastalgia. This condition causes the breasts to become hard and painful and it appears to be an extension of the breast tenderness many women experience before a period. One of the causes can be too high a dose of oestrogen during hormone replacement therapy (HRT). If so, the dose can be adjusted. Another cause may be low levels of essential fatty acids and here a daily dose of evening primrose oil may help – for more in-depth information see my

Quick Guide to Evening Primrose Oil (Boxtree). Evening primrose oil is available on prescription to treat breast pain. Cutting down on caffeine has also been shown to help improve mastalgia, and reduce the risk of non-malignant breast lumps.

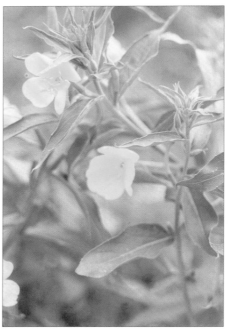

It is also important that we examine our breasts regularly to discover any irregularities as early as possible. One in nine women develop breast cancer and the older we are, the higher the risk. Any lump should be reported without delay to the doctor although only one in ten lumps is discovered to be malignant. Any change in shape or position of the breast, any dimpling, or discharge from the nipple, any lumps in the armpit or collarbone area or any swelling of the upper arm should also be reported to your GP as soon as possible.

DEPRESSION

Few realise the extent to which hormones control us physically and psychologically and many are surprised at how dramatically the menopause can alter the way we feel. During the menopause many women suddenly feel as though they have been stripped of their femininity and sexuality and this can be very depressing. However, this unpleasant symptom can almost always be rectified by maintaining our levels of oestrogen. This can either be achieved through Hormone Replacement Therapy or by eating oestrogen-rich foods (see page 90–1). Taking a daily dose of evening primrose oil may also help to ease depression by naturally balancing the hormones.

HORMONE REPLACEMENT THERAPY

Hormone replacement therapy or HRT has been found to be 98 percent effective in the elimination of both hot flushes and night sweats, as well as improving depression. It is also thought to protect us against osteoporosis and heart disease. However, there is a huge amount of often conflicting advice bombarding women from every side regarding HRT. It doesn't help that many GPs are almost as bewildered as the rest of us. For this reason it may be better to consult one of the special menopause clinics or well women centres if you are thinking of giving HRT a try. Many of the women who try HRT give up within the first year of what could be a long and profitable treatment simply because their GPs have prescribed them an unsuitable dose. The 'standard' prescription can be just the first step in a quite complicated process of trial and adjustment of type and dosage until the most suitable form of HRT is found.

HRT works by supplying the body with the hormones that it ceases to produce during the menopause – oestrogen and progesterone. It was first used in the 1950s for the treatment of hot flushes. The long-term benefits of the therapy gradually became apparent over the next twenty years when it was found that the women who were treated were less subject to osteoporosis and heart disease. Thus it began to be used more directly for these purposes.

HRT can be taken in pill or patch form and must be used properly every day to be effective. Alternatively, an implant eliminates this need, and is particularly suitable for women who have undergone a hysterectomy. The tiny pellet – containing the hormones programmed for slow release – is placed under the skin, often in a GP's surgery under local anaesthetic. The implant can then be forgotten about until menopausal symptoms return (after about six months) when it is then replaced.

SIDE-EFFECTS

Less than 5 percent of women find that they are intolerant to HRT. The main side-effect of HRT can be a very heavy drug-induced monthly bleed which can often be cured by adjusting the dosage. In many cases the bleeds become lighter as time goes by. There is even a combination of pills currently being researched which contain oestrogen and progesterone in such small doses that no bleeding is induced.

Some women may find that they put on weight while on HRT which is particularly difficult to shift. This is because taking oestrogen often encourages the body to store fat on the hips and thighs. Regular exercise and a healthy, low-fat diet can help to guard against this.

THE CANCER QUESTION – THE BIG WORRY

HRT has long been suspected of increasing the risk of breast cancer. However, the general consensus among doctors is that there is no increased risk of breast cancer if HRT is taken for no more than five years. The risk does increase slightly after this. However, it is comforting to know that patients on HRT are carefully monitored and regular mammograms and frequent self-inspections should pick up on any irregularities in the breast as early as is possible.

THE LONG-TERM BENEFITS OF HRT

Apart from the obvious benefits of HRT in eliminating unpleasant hot flushes, night sweats, depression and improving skin and muscle tone, HRT has been found to decrease the risk of heart problems which is a bigger killer of women than breast cancer. The gynaecologist Dr John Studd has concluded from his studies that HRT also prevents the acceleration of bone loss and acts to increase its density.

NATURAL ALTERNATIVES TO HRT

There are some natural ways of increasing our levels of oestrogen and progesterone, such as eating herbs and other foods that are rich sources of hormone-like substances. For example, sage is high in oestrogen, while wild yam, used in Chinese medicine, contains saponin which has a similar effect to progesterone. Extracts from wild yam can be taken orally or as a cream which is applied to the skin to ease some of the symptoms of the menopause. Ginseng, dong quai, black cohosh, and various other herbs and soya products, all of which contain oestrogen-like substances, are also on the market. Sage can even be bought in tincture (liquid extract) form for the express purpose of treating hot flushes. If HRT is not for you, then herbal treatments are worth a try under the guidance of a qualified medical herbalist (see Useful Addresses).

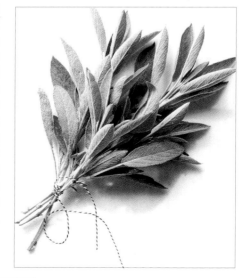

DIET

Diet is extremely important in maintaining strong bones, a healthy heart and glowing skin during the menopause. Follow the healthy eating guidelines laid out in Chapter 1 and cut down on processed foods that are high in fat, sugar or salt.

If you are feeling at a low ebb, your diet may be lacking zinc. This important mineral helps to maintain the body's defence system and is mainly found in seafood, red meat, dairy products and in some green vegetables and cereals.

Menopausal women may also need to increase their intake of certain nutrients if they are on HRT. As a result of the induced monthly bleed, many of the vitamins and minerals present in the blood are lost. Vitamins B12, C and E, folic acid, and iron are all involved in the maintenance of blood systems. Vitamin B12 is found naturally in foods of animal source such as offal, meat, poultry, fish, eggs, milk and cheese. Vitamin C is mainly found in fruit and vegetables while vitamin E is found in vegetable oils, eggs and wholegrains. The richest sources of folic acid are liver, wheatgerm, broccoli and green cabbage and iron is mainly found in red meat and fortified breakfast cereals.

EXERCISE

Regular exercise not only helps us to control our weight, it also helps to maintain a healthy heart and protect us against osteoporosis. Any exercise which really gets your heart and circulation going will do. From a brisk walk for thirty minutes or so three times a week to swimming or tennis and other forms of aerobic exercise. If you would like to join a keep-fit class, low impact aerobics is far better than the high impact variety which can put too much pressure on middle-aged joints. The same goes for jogging – take it easy, wear proper jogging shoes for support and always jog on grass rather than concrete.

If your main form of exercise is swimming, it is important to do some weight-bearing exercise as well as this improves the consistency of our bone and helps prevent osteoporosis. Games like tennis and badminton are excellent, as would be a programme of gentle weight training (not to be confused with weight lifting!). If you belong to a gym, ask the instructor to show you how to use weights or dumb bells. You can buy weighted wrist bands for use at home or even make the movements holding tins of beans! However, you need to be shown how to do the exercises safely to avoid injury.

Seek the advice of your doctor before starting an exercise regime.

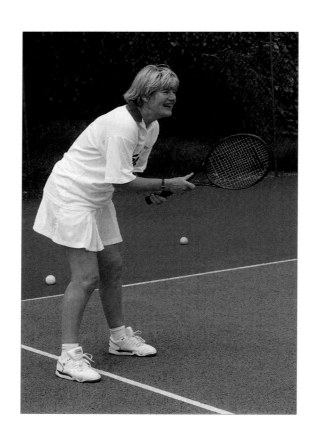

CHAPTER 8

Mature

A geing is inevitable and during our later years our hair turns grey, our skin less elastic, our eyesight deteriorates and we are at the highest risk of disease. However, this is also the time when we possess greater wisdom and are most richly experienced in life. The majority of us will retire from our jobs during our sixties which leaves plenty of time for travel and for doing all the things we have always wanted to do. You may like to learn a foreign language, how to play a musical instrument or something more active, such as golf. Both men and women have taken up scuba-diving or gone on playing high-level tennis well into their later years. The secret is to take things at your own level. Do not forgo the pleasure of learning to play a musical instrument just because you will never get into a symphony orchestra. If your favourite pastimes seem to tire you out, simply take a rest and enjoy them at a slower pace. The key to enjoying our old age is to keep in good health and maintain high energy levels. This can be accomplished through a healthy diet combined with vitamin and mineral supplements to boost our protection against disease, and regular exercise.

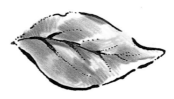

LIFESPAN VERSUS LIFE EXPECTANCY

All species have their own lifespan, which is defined as being the maximum length of time they can live. For human beings this is around 120 years. The difference between maximum lifespan and life expectancy depends upon environmental and genetic factors. In industrialised countries life expectancy had risen to sixty-seven in 1946, and today it stands at around seventy-four. These increases are largely due to improved hygiene conditions preventing bacterial infections. The vast majority die prematurely from degenerative diseases such as heart disease and cancer.

The good news is that we can extend our life expectancy by avoiding foods, habits and situations which increase our risk of developing the biggest killers: heart disease and cancer. By controlling our levels of stress at work and in daily life we can help to maintain our immune system for longer, and by maintaining a keen interest in our friends, family and pastimes we will exercise our minds and stave off mental decline and depression. Exercise is also important to prevent osteoporosis (thinning of the bones – see previous chapter) and protect us against heart disease. These simple lifestyle changes will make our later years some of our most enjoyable ones yet!

WHAT CAUSES AGEING?

In simple terms, there seem to be two types of ageing. The first is the natural, chronological state of growing older which happens to us all. There is not a lot we can do to influence this and, if we are lucky, we can remain fit and active until the end of our lives. The second type is premature, degenerative ageing. This is when we develop diseases such as arthritis and cataracts that so often plague the elderly. Recent research carried out by top scientists around the globe has shown that free radical cell damage is largely responsible for this degenerative ageing.

Free radicals are some of our foremost foes in the ageing process. They are created within us as a result of breathing in oxygen. In small numbers, they are useful in helping our immune system, but problems arise when the body produces too many free radicals. Excessive numbers of free radicals end up damaging our cell walls, causing the protein which holds the body together to disintegrate. Although we are not aware of it happening at the time, the effects of this wholesale destruction of our cells is linked to just about every serious disease in the body including heart disease and cancer. But there are ways in which you can help yourself to better health.

HOW ARE FREE RADICALS FORMED?

Free radicals are produced by oxidation, the same process that causes butter to go rancid when it is left out of the fridge or cars to go rusty when exposed to the air. Although the body itself won't go rusty, its cells are affected in a similar way. This is why free radicals are so damaging. They are continually being produced in the body as an important part of our normal metabolism and in an ideal world they are dealt with by built-in safety mechanisms inside us. However, free radicals are also created by a number of outside influences, such as pollution, which is dramatically spreading in our environment. Our increasing exposure to factors such as pesticides, tobacco smoke, car exhaust systems and ultra-violet radiation from the sun all add up to more free radicals being created than the body was originally designed to cope with.

ANTIOXIDANTS TO THE RESCUE!

It has recently been discovered that antioxidant nutrients present in fruits, vegetables, wholegrains and certain herbs have the power to neutralise free radicals and so prevent cell damage. The key antioxidants are beta-carotene (the inactive or provitamin form of vitamin A), vitamins C and E, selenium, copper, zinc and manganese. Each year new antioxidants are discovered and top-level research around the world shows that these vital nutrients are so powerful that they provide us with the potential to boost our immunity against life-threatening illnesses, prevent serious disorders, such as cataracts, and even reduce the signs of ageing. Prevention is certainly better than cure, and if we ensure that our diet is full of antioxidant nutrients, we can guard against the cell damage that leads to these degenerative illnesses.

Experts state that we need to eat *at least* five portions of fruits and vegetables (excluding potatoes) daily to obtain optimum levels of beta-carotene and vitamin C, but getting hold of vitamin E and selenium, two of the most powerful antioxidants, is not so simple. Vitamin E is mainly found in vegetable oils and you would have to eat, for example, 450g (1lb) of sunflower seeds, more than 2.5kg (5lb) of wheatgerm or drink over 2 litres (4 pints) of corn oil a day to get the same intake of vitamin E found in a common 400IU (International Units) capsule. Selenium occurs naturally in some types of soil and is found in wholegrains and root vegetables and in animals that graze on the soil. However, studies show that on average our daily intake of selenium has dropped from 60mcg a day in 1975 to 35mcg and below today. For these reasons, it may be easier to supplement a healthy diet with the antioxidant vitamins and minerals, which are available together in a tablet or capsule, than to rely on obtaining the levels our bodies require from food. This is particularly important if you smoke or are exposed to high levels of pollution – the most potent creator of free radicals.

CANCER

This disease is frighteningly common and yet there still remains no proven cure. Although we know how cancer can occur, it is still not clear why it affects some and not others. Unfortunately, cases of cancer are on the increase and it is thought that this rise is linked to environmental factors such as pollution. However there have been several encouraging studies carried out throughout the world which clearly show that many types of cancer are largely linked to diet, and in particular to the amounts of antioxidant vitamins in the diet. The rates of cancer vary from country to country depending upon what foods and nutrients are eaten. For example, those living in southern Italy, Spain and Greece are thought to

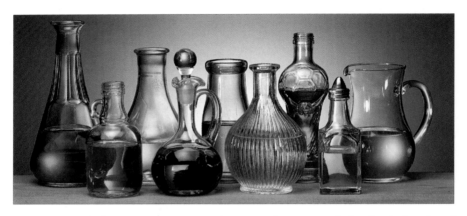

be protected from many types of cancer because of the high levels of antioxidants that they eat. The Mediterranean diet is rich in olive oil (high in vitamin E) and fresh fruits and vegetables (high in beta-carotene and vitamin C), whereas we northern Europeans tend to eat more processed foods and less fresh produce and have a higher risk of cancer and heart disease.

HEART DISEASE

This is the biggest killer of people in Britain and it causes over 160,000 premature deaths every year – well over 3,000 each week! A recent Government health survey found that nine out of ten Britons run a risk of heart disease or strokes – a statistic that the government is anxious to improve considering that heart disease costs the NHS over £500 million each year and takes up over 5,000 hospital beds at any one time. The main risk factors linked to heart disease are smoking, heredity, high cholesterol levels, alcohol, obesity and lack of exercise.

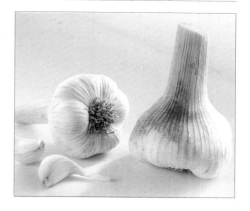

To reduce your risk of developing heart disease, don't smoke or drink to excess and adopt a healthy, low-fat diet as outlined in Chapter 1. Eating plenty of fruits and vegetables will supply your body with the antioxidant nutrients to help combat free radical damage to your cells and reduce your levels of cholesterol. Two of the most important foods to help maintain a healthy heart are garlic and fish oil, such as cod liver oil. Garlic truly is a 'wonder herb'. Not only is it antifungal, antiseptic and a great natural immune-booster, it has been medically proven to reduce cardiovascular problems, especially high blood cholesterol. Garlic tastes great in food, but if you do not like the smell or taste, it is available in odourless capsules.

Cod liver oil is also renowned for its potent smell and taste and for its beneficial effect on heart conditions. It works by increasing the levels of protective cholesterol – high density lipoprotein (HDL). There are good and bad types of cholesterol. A diet high in saturated fat (animal fat) will increase the 'bad' form of cholesterol called low-density lipoprotein (LDL) that encourages deposits in the arteries. Fortunately, our bodies have their own defence mechanism against this, in the form of HDL. It is the job of HDL to keep our cholesterol levels under control and a daily dose of cod liver oil can significantly increase our levels of protective HDL, thereby reducing the risk of heart disease.

ARTHRITIS

During the later years, many find their mobility becomes increasingly restricted by arthritis. This crippling condition is the greatest single cause of disability in Britain and it affects over twenty million people. There are two basic forms of arthritis: the most frequent is osteoarthritis and the less common is rheumatoid arthritis. Osteoarthritis is a 'wear and tear' disorder of the cartilage, associated with changes in the underlying bone which cause joint problems. This usually afflicts the hip, knee and thumb joints. Rheumatoid arthritis is linked to damage to the immune system which is thought to be linked to genetic disorders, diet and certain types of infection. The symptoms of both conditions are inflammation within the joints causing pain, swelling, warmth, redness of overlying skin, joint deformities and restricted mobility.

Diet can play an important role in improving arthritis and many sufferers have reported that their symptoms subside if they switch to a wholefood diet rich in fresh fruit and vegetables and low in processed, refined foods. A study reported in *The Lancet* in 1991 describes how arthritic patients on a one-year vegetarian diet benefited from reduced swelling, greater mobility of the joints and a stronger grip. Cod liver oil has also been shown to effectively reduce the symptoms of arthritis. The essential fatty acids present in cod liver oil produce chemicals – prostaglandins – which reduce inflammation. Cod liver oil also contains vitamin D – a lack of which can cause aches and pains similar to arthritic pains. It is particularly important as we get older to get enough vitamin D through our diet as ageing reduces the skin's ability to manufacture vitamin D from sunlight.

OSTEOPOROSIS

As we get older, our bones get thinner and can become very fragile as a result of osteoporosis (see previous chapter). To help prevent this disease, a daily supplement of magnesium, calcium and vitamin D will help to strengthen our bones.

BRAIN POWER

Senility is not an inevitable part of old age, it is a sign of a diseased mind and a quarter of all senile dementia cases can be cured. Thyroid problems can be the cause of chronic forgetfulness and confusion and this should be medically checked. One of the most distressing problems of old age is Alzheimer's disease. This tragic brain disease causes the elderly to lose their memory and there is currently no way to improve their situation. However, French researchers have shown that some Alzheimer's sufferers have low levels of certain antioxidant vitamins in their bloodstream, which could be a contributory factor. Free radicals damage brain cells much as they do other cells in the body. This may help to explain why the ancient herb ginkgo biloba has been shown to improve memory. Ginkgo biloba is the oldest tree in existence and its leaves contain vitamin C, bioflavonoids and other antioxidants. There have been over 300 studies, mainly in Europe, over the last twenty-five years to establish its actions, particularly its ability to boost blood circulation. Ginkgo biloba extract has been shown to have a particular alliance with brain tissue and it is a licensed medicine in Germany for cerebral insufficiency (poor blood supply to the brain). Cerebral insufficiency is a major cause of senile dementia and the early development of Alzheimer's disease.

WAR ON WRINKLES

As we grow older our skin renews and repairs itself at a much slower pace, while our levels of elastin and collagen that keep skin firm are depleted, resulting in drier, sagging, wrinkled skin. There is little we can do to stop the natural ravages of time on our skin, but there are some simple measures that everyone can take to keep it looking its best for as long as possible.

The most important rule is to stay out of the sun, which is the number one enemy of skin. All dermatologists agree that protecting our skin with a sunblock is one anti-ageing measure that really works. It is also helpful to enrich our diet with vitamins, oils and antioxidants as good skin stems from within. The essential fatty acids found in fish and vegetable oils are vital for healthy skin cells, keeping them moist and strong. However, the most important vitamins for a healthy skin are antioxidants, especially vitamins A, C and E.

Last, but not least, a daily skincare routine involving cleansing and moisturising will help to keep your complexion looking good. The products you use do not need to be expensive or state of the art, but those containing the antioxidant vitamins and active herbal extracts will help to protect your skin against free radical damage and maintain skin softness.

DIET

To make the most of our later years it is important to be fit and healthy and a nutritious diet will boost our natural defences against disease and give us the energy we need to live life to the full. Follow the healthy eating guidelines outlined in Chapter 1 by eating a mainly wholefood diet with lots of fruit and vegetables. Many people find that as they get older their appetite diminishes and they eat a lot less. Other age-related problems, such as impaired mobility, diminished taste and smell, poor dental health and lack of money can also lead to a greatly reduced diet. However, our nutritional needs are at their highest during the later years – so if you are not getting all the nutrients you need from your diet, you should seriously consider taking a daily multivitamin and mineral supplement.

The elderly have increased needs for several vitamins and minerals, especially the antioxidant nutrients. Fruits and vegetables are often the first foods to be cut from our diet as we get older as they tend to require

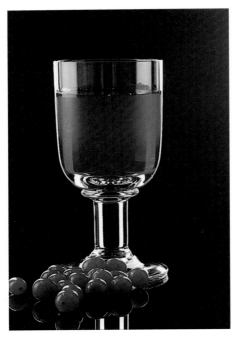

a lot of chewing. If this is a problem for you, choose softer fruits and vegetables and cook them for longer, chop in small pieces or even purée them. Vegetable soups and stews and fresh fruit juices are easier ways to reap the many benefits of their nutritious content.

Some vitamins and minerals are needed to release energy from our food and low levels can lead to tiredness and sometimes even depression. The B-complex vitamins are required to convert the food we eat into energy and vitamins B5 (pantothenic acid) and B6 are also involved in the immune system by helping to form antibodies. Iodine, iron and copper are all involved in energy production, so we need to ensure that we get plenty of these essential nutrients too. Copper also helps to maintain a healthy immune system as does manganese and zinc. Unfortunately, zinc deficiency is common in old age and it has a vital role in healing wounds and maintaining our immune system.

STRETCHING AND MOBILITY EXERCISES

It is essential that we stretch our joints and muscles regularly during the later years, especially if you have arthritis or have suffered an injury that results in stiffness. Any body part that you cannot move through its full normal range of motion needs to be repeatedly stretched so that you can slowly, often over weeks or months, regain full mobility. Gentle exercise can make a big difference to our strength and muscle-tone. One study carried out by Dr Dawn Skelton at the Royal Free Hospital in London found that women aged seventy-five to ninety-three could strengthen their thigh muscles by 25 percent through just three hours of gentle exercise each week for three months. This is the equivalent of setting back our biological clock by sixteen to twenty years! She has written a comprehensive booklet *Exercise for Healthy Ageing* which is published by the charity Research Into Ageing (see Useful Addresses). Some of the basic warm-up and stretching exercises in the booklet are outlined below. Make these a part of your daily routine and you could also feel the benefits of renewed physical strength and mobility.

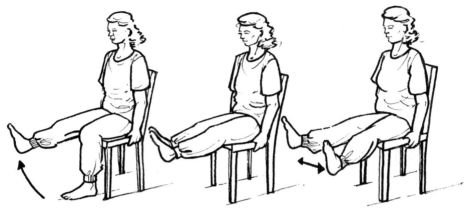

1 Seated, holding on to the sides of the chair, lift one leg, keeping it straight, a few inches off the floor and then lift the other leg to join it. Part the legs about six inches and then bring the legs together and put them down again.

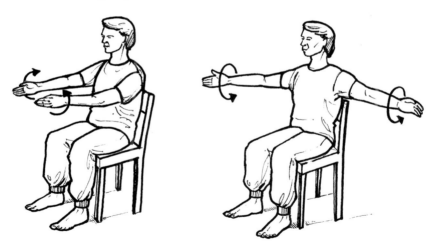

2 Seated, put your arms out in front of you keeping the elbows slightly bent. Move your arms in opposing circular motions. Take them out to the side and repeat.

3 Seated at the front of the chair, keep one leg bent and straighten the other. Place your hands on the bent knee and bend gently forward keeping the back straight. Hold for a slow count of four. Try to go a little further each time.

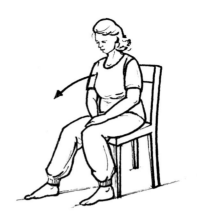

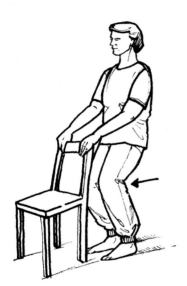

4 Stand with your feet apart and toes forward. Keeping the back upright and heels on the floor, bend the knees slightly. Hold for the count of four, then return to the standing position. Remember not to bend down too far.

5 Standing, with a chair at your side and a hand holding on for support, gently swing your leg forwards and back. Feel the hip moving gently. Change sides and repeat.

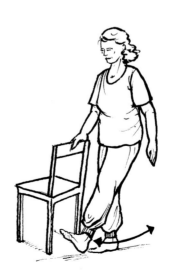

GLOSSARY

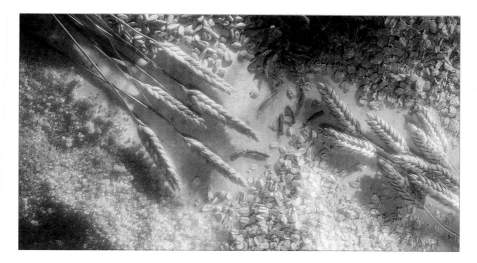

Amino acids – the building-blocks of protein.

Antibiotic – a substance which inhibits the growth of, or destroys, micro-organisms which cause infectious diseases.

Antifungal – a substance which prevents and eliminates fungal infections, e.g. athlete's foot.

Anti-inflammatory – a substance that reduces inflammation of body tissues, so reducing pain and swelling.

Antioxidant – a substance that prevents oxidation. Antioxidant nutrients include beta-carotene, vitamin C and vitamin E.

Antiseptic – a substance which fights infections and germs on the surface of the skin.

Cholesterol – a fatty substance that has many important functions throughout the body. Excess cholesterol may be deposited in the lining of an artery and can limit the flow of blood to the heart.

Degenerative disease – the loss of the capacity of cells, tissues and organs needed for the body to function properly.

Diuretic – a substance that increases the flow of urine by promoting the excretion of salts and water via the kidneys.

Enzyme – a substance produced by the body that regulates biochemical reactions.

Episiotomy – an incision into the tissues surrounding the opening of the vagina during a difficult birth.

Essential fatty acids – unsaturated fatty acids which are converted within the body into larger and more highly unsaturated fatty acids which have important functions in the brains cells and other areas in the body. Some essential fatty acids are converted into prostaglandins. EFAs cannot be formed by the body therefore must be taken in the diet.

Free radical – a reactive particle that contains one or more unpaired electrons, causing it to be highly unstable and sometimes destructive within the body.

Gluten – a mixture of two proteins which is present in wheat, barley, oats and rye and is important for its baking properties. Some people are intolerant to gluten and should avoid these foods.

Heredity – the process whereby our genes are inherited from our parents.

HRT – hormone replacement therapy often prescribed to women during the menopause to provide the hormones oestrogen and progesterone that the body ceases to produce naturally.

Oxidation – the process of using oxygen to release energy from cells. Its side-effect is to produce free radicals.

Perineum – the region of the body from the anus to the urethral opening, through which women urinate.

Pituitary gland – a gland situated in the base of the skull which releases important hormones.

Prolactin – a hormone , synthesised and stored in the pituitary gland, that stimulates milk production after childbirth and also stimulates the production of progesterone.

Prostaglandin – short-lived hormone-like chemicals which regulate the activities of cells in the body.

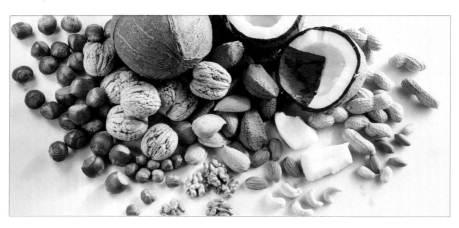

Legumes – beans, pulses, lentils, peas and peanuts – vegetables that are rich in fibre and protein.

Lymphatic drainage system – this part of the immune system interacts with the bloodstream through special ducts and it plays an important role in the removal of waste.

Nervous system – a vast network of cells that carry information in the form of nerve impulses to and from all parts of the body in order to induce body activity.

Osteoporosis – thinning of the bones so that they become fragile and liable to fracture.

Spina bifida – a developmental defect in which the new-born baby has part of the spinal cord exposed through a gap in the backbone. The symptoms may include paralysis of the legs and mental retardation.

Thrombosis – a condition in which the blood becomes thick and sticky and forms a blood clot which can lead to a heart attack.

Thyroid gland – situated in the base of the neck, this gland regulates the body's metabolic rate by the secretion of thyroid hormone.

USEFUL ADDRESSES

Breast Cancer Care
Kiln House
210 New King's Road
London SW6 4NZ
Helpline: 0500 245 345
Specialises in all aspects of breast cancer care.

British Heart Foundation
14 Fitzhardinge Street
London W1H 4DH
Tel: 0171 935 0185
Send an SAE for information on prevention of heart disease and all aspects of heart problems.

British Homoeopathic Association
27a Devonshire Street
London W1N 1RJ
Tel: 0171-935 2163
Send an SAE for a list of registered practitioners in your area.

Carer's National Association
Ruth Pitter House
20/25 Glasshouse Yard
London EC1A 4JS
Helpline: 0171-490 8818
They will put carers in touch with local support groups and can give advice on how to get respite care, what financial benefits are available, how to apply for them and all other aspects of caring for the elderly or disabled in the home.

CRY-SIS Support Group
BM CRY-SIS
London WC1N 3XX
Tel: 0171-404 5011
Daily, 8am–11pm
Provides support and advice to parents of babies who cry incessantly or have sleep problems.

Evening Primrose Oil Office
Tel: 0171-720 8596
Telephone for further information on evening primrose oil.

Folic Acid Helpline
Tel: 0181-994 9874
Monday–Friday, 2pm–10pm

Foresight
The Association for the Promotion of Preconceptual Care
28 The Paddock
Godalming
Surrey GU7 1XD
Send an SAE for dietary and other preconceptual information.

Henry Doubleday Research Association
Ryton Organic Gardens
Ryton-on-Dunsmore
Coventry CV8 3LG
Tel: 01203 303517
Largest organisation of organic gardeners in the world and new members are welcome. Products and gardening books available by mail-order. Can also advise on local organic produce suppliers.

Institute for Complementary Medicine
PO Box 194
London SE16 1QZ
Tel: 0171-237 5165
Send an SAE for further information on complementary therapies.

Institute of Optimum Nutrition (ION)
13 Blades Court
Deodar Road
London SW15 2NU
Tel: 0181 877 9993
An independent educational trust which aims to promote health through optimum nutrition. ION organises courses, seminars and consultations and has an extensive library of books on nutrition. Yearly membership of ClubION (costing £9) entitles you to receive Optimum Nutrition Magazine *quarterly as well as a 10 percent discount on courses, books and seminars.*

International Federation of Aromatherapists
Stanford House
2/4 Chiswick High Road
London W4 1TH
Tel: 0181-742 2605
*Send an SAE for a list of registered practitioners
in your area.*

La Lèche League of Great Britain
BM 3424
London WC1N 3XX
Tel: 0171-242 1278 (24-hour answerphone)

Margaret Pyke Centre
15 Bateman's Buildings
Soho Square
London W1V 6JB
Tel: 0171-734 9351
*Offer complete assessment for suitability for
HRT and the necessary medication. No need for
referral by a GP and no charge except for
prescriptions, although donations are welcomed
as this organisation relies on voluntary
contributions.*

Marie Stopes Centre
108 Whitfield Street
London W1P 6BE
Tel: 0171-388 2585
(and also in Leeds and Manchester)
*Offer a fifty-minute 'Menocheck' to assess
hormone levels, general health and suitability
for HRT. There is no need for referral by a GP
but there is a charge of £100 for the check-up
and for any prescriptions.*

**National Association for Premenstrual
Syndrome (NAPS)**
PO Box 72
Sevenoaks
Kent TN13 1XQ
Information line: 01732 741709

National Childbirth Trust (NCT)
Alexandra House
Oldham Terrace
London W3 6NH
Tel: 0181-992 8637

National Institute of Medical Herbalists
56 Longbrook Street
Exeter EX4 6AH
Tel: 01392 426022
*Monday–Friday, 1.30pm–5 pm
Send an SAE for a list of registered practitioners
in your area.*

National Osteoporosis Society
PO Box 10
Radstock
Bath BA3 3YB
Tel: 01761 471 771
Send an SAE for information.

Quit
Victory House
170 Tottenham Court Road
London W1P 0HA
Tel: 0800 00 22 00
*Daily 9.30am–5.30pm
A helpline to give support to those wishing to
break the smoking habit.*

Research Into Ageing
Baird Street
15–17 St Cross Street
London EC1N 8UN
Tel: 0171-404 6878
*Research Into Ageing is a national medical
research charity committed to improving the
health and quality of life of older people. It has
published a comprehensive booklet on* Exercise
for Healthy Ageing *written by Dr Dawn
Skelton who has carried out many studies on
exercise and the elderly. The booklet contains
over thirty-five exercises devised by experts
specifically for the elderly. It costs £3 and is
available by mail-order from the above address.
For more information about Research Into
Ageing or to make a donation, write to the
above address.*

**Society for the Promotion of Nutritional
Therapy (SPNT)**
PO Box 47
Heathfield
East Sussex TN21 8ZX
Tel: 01435 867007
*Send an SAE for more information and details
of their nutritional bulletins.*

Soil Association
86 Colston Street
Bristol BS1 5BB
Tel: 0117-929 0661
*Their symbol is a consumer guarantee that food
is high quality and genuinely organically grown.
The Soil Association welcomes new members
and can also advise on stockists of organically
grown produce.*

Vegetarian Society
Parkdale
Dunham Road
Altrincham
Cheshire WA14 4QG
Tel: 0161-928 0793

**Woman's Nationwide Cancer Control
Campaign**
Helpline: 0171-729 2229
*They will answer any questions on cancer, its
diagnosis, treatment and aftercare, etc.*

SUPPLIERS OF NATURAL REMEDIES

The following all offer a mail-order service:

Aromatherapy Associates
68 Maltings Place
Bagleys Lane
London SW6 2BY
Tel: 0171-731 8129
Suppliers of essential oil blends.

Dr Edward Bach Centre
Mount Vernon
Wallingford
Oxon OX10 0PZ
Tel: 01491 834678
Suppliers of the Bach Flower Remedies.

G Baldwin & Co
171–173 Walworth Road
London SE17 1RW
Tel: 0171-703 5550
Suppliers of herbs/essential oils.

MENSTRUAL CHART

	Jan	Feb	Mar	Apr	May	June	July	Aug	Sep	Oct	Nov	Dec
NAME						YEAR						

	Jan	Feb	Mar	Apr	May	June	July	Aug	Sep	Oct	Nov	Dec
1												
2												
3												
4												
5												
6												
7												
8												
9												
10												
11												
12												
13												
14												
15												
16												
17												
18												
19												
20												
21												
22												
23												
24												
25												
26												
27												
28												
29												
30												
31												

SUGGESTED KEY TO SYMBOLS:

M (or red line) = Menstruation
B = Breat tenderness
W = Fluid retention
I = Irritability

P = Panic attack
A = Asthma attack
D = Depression
H = Headache

INDEX

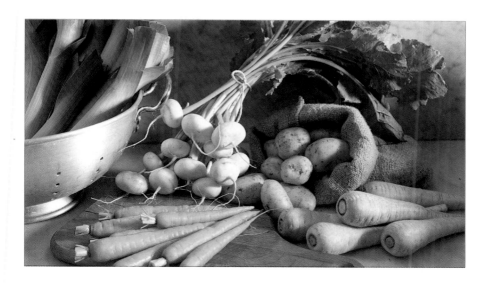

PICTURE CREDITS

Anthony Blake Photo Library: pp12, 25, 30, 33, 34, 60, 100, Heather Brown p103,
Gerrit Buntrock pp28, 36, 109, James Duncan p41, Merehurst Limited p59, Milk Marque p32,
No Cookbooks/Stockfood p36, Graham Parish p96,
Rosenfeld Images Ltd pp5, 11, 14, 17, 29, 61, 62, 86, 90, 97, 104,
Charlie Stebbings p13, Jane Stockman p74.

Concept at Charles Barker pp52, 82, 88.

Sally & Richard Greenhill Photo Library pp8, 21, 44, 45, 46, 56, 67, 68, 69, 72, 77, 79, 92.

Health Education Authority p14.

Raymond Turvey p23.

HOW TO ORDER YOUR BOXTREE BOOKS BY LIZ EARLE

LIZ EARLE'S QUICK GUIDES

Available Now

☐	0 7522 1631 7	Acne	£3.99
☐	0 7522 1663 5	Antioxidants	£3.99
☐	1 85283 542 7	Aromatherapy	£3.99
☐	1 85283 544 3	Baby and Toddler Foods	£3.99
☐	0 7522 1645 7	Beating Cellulite	£3.99
☐	0 7522 1668 6	Beating PMS	£3.99
☐	0 7522 1641 4	Cod Liver Oil	£3.99
☐	1 85283 979 1	Detox	£3.99
☐	0 7522 1636 8	Dry Skin and Eczema	£3.99
☐	0 7522 1619 8	Evening Primrose Oil	£3.99
☐	0 7522 1675 9	Food Allergies	£3.99
☐	0 7522 1673 2	Food Combining	£3.99
☐	1 85283 543 5	Food Facts	£3.99
☐	0 7522 1635 X	Hair Loss	£3.99
☐	0 7522 1685 6	Healthy Menopause	£3.99
☐	0 7522 1680 5	Healthy Pregnancy	£3.99
☐	0 7522 1614 7	Herbs for Health	£3.99
☐	0 7522 1626 0	Juicing	£3.99
☐	0 7522 1690 2	Post-natal Health	£3.99
☐	1 85283 984 8	Successful Slimming	£3.99
☐	1 85283 546 X	Vegetarian Cookery	£3.99
☐	1 85283 989 9	Vitamins and Minerals	£3.99
☐	0 7522 1636 8	Youthful Skin	£3.99
☐	1 85283 518 4	Liz Earle's Ace Plan The New Guide to Super Vitamins A, C and E	£4.99
☐	1 85283 554 0	Liz Earle's Ace Plan – Weight-Loss for Life	£4.99
☐	0 7522 1699 6	Liz Earle's Bikini Diet	£4.99

All these books are available at your local bookshop or can be ordered direct from the publisher. Just tick the titles you want and fill in the form. Prices and availability subject to change without notice.

Boxtree Cash Sales, PO Box 11, Falmouth, Cornwall TR10 9EN

Please send cheque or postal order for the value of the book, and add the following for postage and packing: **UK including BFPO –** £1.00 for one book, plus 50p for the second book, and 30p for each additional book ordered up to a £3.00 maximum. **Overseas including Eire –** £2.00 for the first book, plus £1.00 for the second book, and 50p for each additional book ordered.

OR please debit this amount from my Access/Visa Card (delete as appropriate)

Card number ___ ___ ___ ___ ___ ___ ___ ___ ___ ___ ___ ___ ___ ___ ___ ___

Amount £ .... Expiry date on card ....

Name .... Signed ....

Address ....

....